D1617229

3-23-77

The Time of
Their Dying

The Time of
Their Dying

BY

Stephen S. Rosenfeld

W · W · NORTON & COMPANY · INC · NEW YORK

Library of Congress Cataloging in Publication Data
Rosenfeld, Stephen.
    The time of their dying.
    1. Cancer—Biography.   2. Rosenfeld, Jay C.
3. Rosenfeld, Elizabeth K., 1905 or 6–1976.
I. Title.
RC263.R639   1977   363.1'9'699409 [B]   77–23264

ISBN 0 393 08771 9

2 3 4 5 6 7 8 9 0

To Barbara

Contents

The Time of
Their Dying

Introduction

MY FATHER, Jay C. Rosenfeld, died of cancer at age eighty on October 21, 1975, and my mother, Elizabeth K. Rosenfeld, died, also of cancer, at age seventy on March 25, 1976. They lived long and good lives, and they died long and hard deaths. As they fell ill, really for the first time in their lives, I realized that though I was a mature adult with more than average pretensions to knowledge of the world, I was coming into a new room whose dimensions, lighting, furniture were strange and even awesome to me. I saw that it was possible to live in a century in which death has been dealt out by men on a scale never before contemplated, and to work in a business, newspapering, in which death is a routine part of the job (I broke in, the typical cub, on obits), and yet to have seen death only at a distance denying a true, felt knowledge of it.

When I did get close to death, that of my parents, I found that the sense of it touched and then pervaded my relationship with them and, as time went on, began to color my attitude towards others, making me more impatient to engage in relationships lacking a substantial quotient of personal meaning, or at least fun. There was, I knew, nothing particularly "new" or unusual about either my attitude towards my parents or my attitude towards other people. But—here is my point— neither the culture nor my friends nor my own pattern of reading had informed me that changes of these kinds were in store.

The more I thought about it, the better I understood that my experience, far from being unique, was virtually universal, at least for that privileged minority of the world's inhabitants for whom a general preoccupation with sheer daily survival does not render a special concern for the process of dying a luxury. Modern circumstances have made it the rule, as Sissela Bok has observed, that the leading causes of death are no longer the major communicable diseases but the chronic degenerative diseases which tend to arise much later in life— and, one might add, to develop relatively slowly.

This means that most children will be grown and independent by the time their parents age, fall sick, and die. Indeed, the death of parents now commonly occurs in the context of three generations, since the children of sick and dying parents already will have their own children. Family dependence will almost invariably have been reversed, in a symbolic sense anyway: from the child depending on the parent, the parent comes to depend on the child. And apart from dependence, the death of parents can occasion the final readjustment of a child-parent relationship last calibrated when the child was, say, twenty, and just quitting the nest for a career and family of his own.

In brief, there is an extraordinary opportunity for the exploration of personal avenues of a sort unimagined before. At least that was the way it was for me. It made the time of my parents' dying sad but rich as well.

As it happened, I spent a rather considerable amount of time with them in that period—on leaves from my work, on vacations, on quick weekend trips, and the like. I did this out of a mix of love, duty, and absorption in the process that was going on in their life and in mine. Putting in that time shaped the quality of my life for the two-year period of their travail. Moreover, my family and friends and many others became in their separate ways part of what was happening, since I either shared it explicitly with them or, often, acted implicitly in a way reflecting or testing my developing consciousness of death.

While I was in my twenties and thirties, I had not

considered death—it seemed far from my parents and far from me. "Ah no, the bliss youth dreams is one/For daylight, for the cheerful sun," Matthew Arnold wrote. Now that I am in my mid-forties, I find that I and almost everyone of my generation are acutely conscious of it. People my age can be readier to share accounts of their failing parents than to tell and hear the more familiar stories of their growing children. We are sobered by the parents' ordeal and by our response to it and, not least, by its foretelling of our own fate.

My own account has no particular drama or heroism. That makes it, I think, more relevant and accessible to others, not less. Most of us live ordinary lives, and die ordinary deaths. But in the ordinary there is a range of feeling and detail that is like the pattern in marble, only partly visible on the surface, but penetrating unseen into the body of the stone.

There are no great revelations in this story, though there are some things that, before they were written, I did not relate even to my wife. I have no secrets from her but the circumstances in which disclosure seemed appropriate to the event and to my mood simply did not materialize until now. Further, I have no familial or psychological scores to settle, or none of which I am aware, anyway. With an intent to respect their privacy, I chose to make this my account and not that of my two brothers and my sister, who, as in all families, heard their own tones.

It was, I believe, the emotional and psychological vitality released in the period of my parents' dying that stirred me to undertake a book about it—about the process of their dying, rather than strictly about them. For while they were to me individuals whom I loved and enjoyed, it was not so much of their lives that I wanted to tell as of the manner of their dying and of my involvement then with them. I harbor, too, the hope that other children can come to see the special potential of their situation as their own parents' lives draw to an end.

ONE

Tennis

TENNIS WAS our family game. We had a court, set on a
niche which had been cut into the side of South Mountain at roof level just up the slope from our house. The
roof, in fact, was virtually the only structure visible
from the court. One could look out ten and twenty
miles up the Housatonic River valley in which Pittsfield
sits, toward Mt. Greylock (at 3,505 feet Massachusetts'
highest peak, as every Berkshire County schoolboy
learned), and imagine that our place was a special preserve. Beyond the court, "the woods," our childhood
haunt, stretched back for miles.

As children the four of us regularly climbed the pine tree at the west end of the court, in which one could swiftly disappear from view from the ground and take a hidden perch to watch a tennis game or to gaze at the soft blur of the horizon. Sometimes we ate lunch in the tree, sitting on a board nailed into place years before by the son of the family whose house across South Mountain Road my father had screened off by planted pines. In time, we replaced the wooden swing that had been rigged on chains in our own early years, with a rubber swing seat for our own children, my parents' eleven grandchildren, who were annually in successive attendance through the summer.

Under the tree it was quiet and cool, like a green private room, and sometimes our kids, halting the usual tumult and carnage, would slow as though they had caught the magic themselves.

"Regardez les petites," my father would say to my mother, stopping in mid-game and nodding at the grandchildren.

"Posmotri na detyei," Barbara or I, using Russian, our child-proof language, would say.

The house was being built when my twin brother and I were born in 1932. Later it pleased my father immensely to reap credit for having conceived and executed such a veritable Shangri-la. The place was not only a badge of the comfort and status of someone whose father had been, in his luckier years, a struggling shopkeeper. The court in particular marked his determination to be independent of the nearby Pittsfield Country Club, which, until it could no longer afford such a policy, accepted only one Jewish family.

Squire's pride notwithstanding, my father always regarded some part of the maintenance of the place as the duty of the children. We were brought up on a stiff diet of yard work, a regime I found onerous, absorbing, and character-building in turn. To the end of the time he and my mother lived there, I and sometimes others of the Rosenfeld children would, on vacations, weed out the grass constantly seeping like green ink through the wire fence into the tennis court. The weeding seemed to reestablish a rhythm of family duty, and to freshen our commitment to the soft beauty of the place. It was a token return on what my father and mother had put in.

In those later years my father never actually asked me to go at the grass. But when I stayed up there after a game, working in a slow-moving squat until my legs ached and coming down late for lunch on the terrace, the mildness of his reproof expressed his satisfaction. It made me grimace, though I knew better, that our oldest son, who was no more diligent at nine or ten than I had been, treated my requests for his help as a court weeder with the same impatience that he displayed towards chores at our Virginia home.

To himself my father reserved one chore—cutting the brush which pushed up around the smaller pines planted along either side of the court. I remember him walking, bent, up the curving path from the house, tennis racket in one hand, brush cutter in the other. He took as much pleasure from laying a cluster of alder branches flat on the ground as he did from leaning, as though flicking sugar with tongs, to drop his favorite backhand dump shot over the net.

Cutting brush is one of the more satisfying yard jobs: the butts look clean and the brush itself can be piled in impressive bulk. Recalling how the family used to tease my father for ever being on the prowl with his brush cutter, I have often wandered outside our own tame suburban half-acre in northern Virginia wishing there were more brush to cut. One of our twins, Michael—on his own, I'm sure—often asks if he can cut some brush. The reappearance of this trivial family pattern startles me. On one level I lay it to Michael's industry and good hand-eye coordination; on another level, to a nice fate.

Neither my parents nor any of us children were ever particularly good tennis players. But we played energetically, in and out of different family combinations, for the forty-odd years that my parents lived on South Mountain Road. The memory of their willingness to hit balls back to us when we were kids helped keep me, when I acquired my own four children, ready to hit with them.

At that point, Barbara and I were coming up to Pittsfield for a week or so in the summer before or after our own family vacation elsewhere in New England. That vacation of our own we planned, not without certain misgivings, as the one period in the year when we were thrown as a family entirely upon ourselves, without the distraction of job or school or the complication—better, the simplification—of accommodating to anyone else. For Pittsfield was simple for us. Someone else cooked, there was a pool as well as a court right there, the grandparents indulged the grandchildren and took a lot of the daily routine off Barbara's and my hands.

My parents had the stamina to play only with Barbara and me, not with our children. Though she and I were, unsurprisingly, harder hitters and better players, we nonetheless settled into a regular match of the generations, at my father's bidding, rather than switching partners to even out the sides. Sometimes I wondered if it was because my father wanted to beat us. More likely he wanted to lose—for the symbolic assurance it provided that he had raised a family well. In fact, because Barbara and I tended to play below our level against their soft hits, they sometimes did win.

"You let us," my mother would say reprovingly, ever her children's booster.

"We beat them," my father insisted, giving no verbal quarter.

My father stood in the far corners to serve and used an old-fashioned rocking motion. He hit ground strokes flat-footed and, in his later years, displayed a wiliness only occasionally abandoned for the smashes, now usually misses, of his younger game.

"Your father is very sly," my mother would say to us. "Good shot, Jay."

To the end, he enjoyed tennis enough to curse his own bad shots. He was something of a fanatic about working up a sweat, which I found strange until I got old enough to realize how sweat in sport is welcome evidence of a capacity for self-exertion.

My mother's game reflected her great nervous energy, a family legend. For years we made fun of her serve: a ferociously fast windup, a pause dissipating all its effect, and a flat tap. She had a steady pushed backhand and ran like a rat for any shot within sight. "There's life in the old girl yet," my father said, hundreds of times. Doubles was their game.

Our matches became, I suppose, a family statement. The balls I hit at my mother I hoped she'd hit back. Not scoring points but keeping her in the game was what it was about. With her the ball went back and forth, often with calls of mutual congratulation traded across the net. That was the kind of relationship I had with her.

With my father the play had an edge. He who had done his best to hit balls to me as a boy now tried to hit past me as a man. I would start by holding back out of deference to his age but then would lunge forward with the triple compulsion of exercise, shot making, and competition that all tennis lovers know. I felt, too, there was no reason why he should beat me. I was a good friend of his by this time. The more limited father-adolescent son tension typical of the 1940s, and the reserve with which we had cushioned our different outlooks and styles as I got older, had yielded to a rather mellow family feeling. We could talk easily. But in a sense our tennis was better than conversation. It allowed for the expression of generational hesitancies that had lingered on.

Across the net the two of them would mutter about strategy in between points, my father in the general's role. My consciousness raised by women's lib, I had stopped offering my own wife that kind of advice. But I did something else. I have always found Barbara particularly appealing in a tennis dress and I would approach her after a point. "You are a very sexy person," I might quietly put in, knowing that my father, an old-fashioned person in this area, would not have approved. In the very first quotation, copied in 1914 into the first of his scores of commonplace books, he had quoted Longfellow's lines, "Let not the illusion of thy senses, / Betray thee to deadly offenses"!

Barbara, catching my point with a net player's quickness, would reply in kind.

In August of 1974 we played our last family game. During the preceding May my father had undergone his first operation, for cancer of the prostate—not an unusual operation, nor necessarily a difficult one, for a man of seventy-eight. He had always prided himself on keeping his weight steady, on eating carefully and on exercising regularly, and he snapped back smartly. All of us were slightly incredulous but we thought it simply marvelous that he was back on the court so soon.

Gingerly, adjusting his customary horse-collar-style towel, he tested his step and swing. My mother, hesitant at first to let him play, yielded to his flooding confidence and threw herself into the game. Barbara and I held back a bit but the game went ahead. Barbara hit a medium hard shot up the middle. My father lumbered up from the baseline with his racket extended, intent on the ball. He caught one foot behind the other—the frame is frozen in my mind—and popped up in the air, almost hanging there. His mouth stayed open and his hand went out and he dropped like a statue to the red clay with nothing breaking his fall. A big *oomph* came out and he lay still. The ball rolled to the fence.

The family had often repeated in jest one of my father's old lines, a line he meant seriously. He wanted to die of a heart attack on the tennis court, he had said. I thought—we all thought—that this was the end for him right there. My mind raced back to the image of the one dead body I had previously seen: that of a heavy elderly woman who had collapsed in the lobby of Constitution Hall coming in out of that fantastic snowstorm on the eve of John Kennedy's inaugural. ("What's her name, what's her name?" my editor had screamed on the phone—I didn't know.) My father lay there, lumpy, cheek in the dirt. I felt breathless but oddly relieved. This was the way he had wanted to go.

He wasn't dead, though later, as cancer devoured him, he said he wished he had died then. He was just briefly in shock without wind. Barbara and I ran to him. We undraped his limbs, laid him out like a squirrel pelt on his back, put something under his head, shaded him, and waited for his breath, color, and speech to return.

"Jay," said Barbara, "you gave us quite a scare."

"Dad, you lost the point," I said.

My mother, very quiet, touched his brow and assured him he would soon be all right.

As we later found out, he had two cracked ribs, something of a trophy for a cancer patient of seventy-eight, we felt. Meanwhile, his side ached. Barbara and I lifted him up. My mother brushed off the dirt. We took his arm and walked him down the curving path, through the little orchard in which grew the tasty sickle pears he pridefully picked each year, down the stone steps which we boys had set unevenly into the hill years before and which he had never hired more skilled hands to level. He looked drawn and scared beyond the measure of the bruises.

A year later, in August 1975, Barbara and I, abandoning our usual "private" vacation, took a cottage on

Stockbridge Bowl ten miles down-county for the whole three weeks available to us. My mother murmured apologies for not taking us into the Pittsfield house. But she knew that the racket of the kids would have been too much for my father, and too much for her as well. She needed to be able to concentrate on him.

Every morning we came up from Stockbridge to Pittsfield, and Barbara and I played singles. I had taken weekly lessons, my first ever, for the two preceding months and was delighted, often noisily so, at the improvement in my game, especially the backhand. Barbara, playing up to my game, had never played better. I was acutely conscious of the contrast between the vigor on the court and the decay in the house. My father's bedroom window was almost at eye level from the court and in between strokes I would shoot glances at it, not being able to see into the dark within but thinking that my father could at least hear the pop of the balls.

Did the noise bother him? We asked every day. He nodded no. Our kids, the four of them, wanted to play, too. Sometimes I played with one at a time, sometimes with all four, keeping two or three balls going at once— easier than it sounds because they so often missed. The kids would cry out or groan, and argue about whose turn it was and how long the other had played. I knew these sounds were drifting into my father's window. I felt it was the children's deathbed gift to him.

In March 1975 my mother had undergone her own

first cancer operation. A section of the colon was removed. "Extensive involvement" of the liver had been found. She had lost nearly twenty pounds. But she regained her strength steadily. Chemotherapy was proceeding. As she rose, my father fell. The lines intersected late in the spring. By August, the period of our Berkshire vacation, she was caring for my father virtually around the clock.

Skiing a few winters earlier at Bousquet's, a mile from the house, she had fallen hard on the hill and had been transported down on a toboggan stretcher. The doctor, a young man who did not know her, was confounded to hear her say from the toboggan, "I've got to get up to play tennis"—indoors, on her and my father's faithful winter schedule. And she trotted off. We loved telling that story. She loved hearing it played back. She loved disparaging our boasts about her energy and determination. So when she suddenly appeared unannounced on the court on one of those August mornings, we were startled but not entirely so.

"Bethie," said Barbara. "Children, look who's here."

Her tennis dress hung loosely. It was hot but she wore a sweater. We reclaimed her racket from a child. "I just want to hit for a while," she said.

With Barbara she got on on one side, and I got on the other. I hit carefully, almost as though ladling. "Don't spare your old gray mère," she would have said in other years when someone served up pat balls. She said noth-

27

ing now. She had her old forehand swing, hit with racket folding over quickly to produce a top spin; her backhand was the same old Ping-Pong push shot. But though the strokes were there, the force was not. Her balls just dribbled over, if that.

"Take it easy, Bethie," Barbara said.

It occured to me that she was playing right up to the edge of her by now much-reduced physical limits. I wondered if she should be playing at all. She half ran a few steps.

"Mother," I said.

"Your father," she said, laboring, "needs me." She left the court.

In November 1975—my father had died in October—my mother had a little heart attack. One night some weeks later we phoned from Washington. "I'm feeling better," she said. "I expect to play tennis in the spring."

"You'll win the Davis Cup," I said.

She kept her racket, and my father's, in the corner of the downstairs hall, where tennis gear had always been stowed, until she died the following March.

TWO

First Word

IT DIDN'T TOUCH ME that my parents could die until my father's right hip stiffened painfully while he and my mother were vacationing in London in May 1974 and they chose, with a purposefulness I did not immediately comprehend, to fly home quickly rather than to stay and cope with it abroad. Later I realized how sound was the instinct that took them back to a familiar setting at a moment when they sensed trouble. At the time, knowing how they loved their trips to Paris and London, cities where they sank easily into a decades-old vacation routine of walking, dining, and attending plays and concerts, I thought that something very serious must have happened to make them break off their holiday.

Something very serious had happened, or begun to happen. The cancer which was eventually to kill my father was starting to prowl. But since his first operation was a relatively minor one, for a cancer of the prostate, and since he recovered promptly and without visible complications, we—his children and children-in-law (eight of us)—passed swiftly out of our state of incipient alarm. A clear picture of death requires a long exposure, I was to learn. A sudden snapshot reveals practically nothing at all.

Looking back, I marvel at the extent to which family protectiveness and circumstance had spared me virtually all awareness of death or, for that matter, of other sorts of tragedy until I was almost out of my teens. I was born the year before Hitler came to power and bar mitzvahed the year World War II ended but through that period I never realized that millions were dying in the camps and on the battlefield. It simply was not discussed in the house. The "news," as I recall it, was of struggle and heroism and victory, but not of death.

My father, forty-six (and a World War I combat veteran) at the time of Pearl Harbor, volunteered for the Quartermaster Corps but was turned down. A cousin's husband was badly wounded in the Battle of the Bulge but returned nonetheless, whole and healthy. A family friend who was a doctor sent my brother and me rings made of metal from a downed German plane.

In Sunday School, as it was then called—not, as now, the more ethnically assertive Religious School—it was the time-dimmed travails of Jews in centuries past that filled out the curriculum. American Reform Jews of the war period evidently were not prepared to concede, or at least to hint to their children, that their kin's gamble of seeking safety as a minority within an "advanced" Western society had failed so catastrophically. My sister Jayn actually was born on "Crystal Night," November 10, 1938, the night of a huge Nazi assault on the Jewish community of Germany. Characteristically, or so I later thought, my father kept the news from my mother so as not to upset her.

We had no relatives in Europe to take in or mourn. My father had lost track of his family in Germany decades earlier, and my mother, arriving as an infant from Lithuania and soon orphaned, never even knew the name of the town where she was born.

On a personal level, things were hardly different. All four of my grandparents had died before my brother and I were born. A few relatives who had never been part of our life in Pittsfield passed away at a distance, emotional and geographical. The first person I knew who died was a casual friend a year or two older who was killed in a car crash driving home from a date. In the Marine Corps, in which I served two peacetime years upon graduation from Harvard in 1953, two fellows in my battalion died of—it was said—heat stroke. But I did not know them, since we had been assigned companies by alphabet and their names began with letters far from R.

The only prior death I had observed with some special sadness, though at a physical remove, was that of my aunt Ruby, my father's older sister, whose long decline I tracked chiefly through his somewhat peeved and self-pitying reports. As titular head of the Rosenfeld family and as a near neighbor of Ruby, he called on her every day for years, heard out her complaints about her pains, and went home to mumble to my mother how narrow and self-centered Ruby's concerns were. He must have been scared that it would be that way for him. "I want to go like *that*," he told my mother, snapping his fingers and emphasizing the last word. Otherwise, apart from Ruby, death meant little to me. I cite this record in some awe at the innocence of a twentieth-century man.

My father, however, like many older men, had come increasingly to walk around, and to talk around, the dread subject. "If I should kick out in the near future," he wrote to me six years before his death—he never used the word "die" in speaking of himself—then his estate would work out one way. "If on the other hand the Lord plays a trick on me and grants me longer life," then it would work out another way.

For years he reviewed the ways in which he intended to conserve his assets for his heirs. It was a mild obsession with him, going beyond his businessman's adversary relationship with the tax collector and beyond normal considerations of family prudence. I suppose estate planning is a way of coming to terms with one's eventual passing—a good medium in which to practice dying, so to speak. My father even threw in a little of his gentle nineteenth-century sexism. "Mama," he wrote in another estate dissertation, "does not like to discuss these things but I feel that they should be disseminated. We can pray that it may not be necessary to apply any plans for a long time but when a man passes seventy-three he has few delusions or, for that matter, fears."

I'm not so sure of delusions but I think at that point he had a lot of fears. He was retired, living well, enjoying good health, engaged in various activities that pleased him, surrounded by family and friends: he did not want to die.

Sometimes I felt impatience towards his circumlocutions and labored style, no different in speech than in letters. Only later did I learn to respect the impulse that made him want to move towards death in a verbal manner, as in a legal-estate manner, of his own choosing. From being stiffened by his rhetoric, I became softened by awareness of his fear.

Every morning he bought the *New York Times* "upstreet" in the center of Pittsfield two miles away, and every afternoon he plucked Pittsfield's own *Berkshire Eagle* out of the mailbox at the foot of the driveway 100 yards down—the paper boy would shut the mailbox door to signal that the paper was there. At once he turned to the obituary page, remarking to whoever was listening on the ages and circumstances of people younger than himself who had died.

When friends of his were written up, he would sit in silence and gaze off, perhaps recall a particular scene or characteristic, or produce some capsule evaluation of the person's life. "I knew her on Francis Avenue," he might say, alluding, as he always did, with a studied sense of social equality, to the old working-class neighborhood where he had grown up before World War I. "With everything he had, he had nothing," he once said of an old friend who had died rich but separated from his family. At those moments he seemed to be writing his own obituary, scanning the equation of his own life.

Little given to such moralistic weighings, my mother tended to confine herself to murmuring sympathy for those who survived. I don't think she was necessarily anticipating her own bereavement when my father died first, as she (almost eleven years younger) surely expected him to do. Rather, she seemed to be recalling her own circumstances upon being orphaned in New York as a child of eight years.

My father had known at least some of his grandparents; he was a grown man when his own parents died; he had a brother and sister and various cousins, most of them with their own families. Not only did my mother lose her own parents early; but her two sisters, both married, had no children. He came from a thick family context, she from a thin one. To my father, taking his context for granted, death was an occasion for community judgment; to my mother, it was more a time of personal loneliness.

She never evinced any concern about her own future death. When he brought up the matter of his, she would say, "Jay, let's not talk of that."

And so it was a shock, an absolute shock, when toward the end of a gray, rainy afternoon in March 1975 I received a phone call in my office from one of her doctors in Pittsfield. I forget who. She had developed cancer of the liver, I understood him to say; she had been operated on earlier that day, and would be treated, but the prognosis was poor.

I gasped, and not only at what this meant for her. I not only had expected but had counted on my father's dying first. That was the order of the family universe. Not just by virtue of her being ten years younger than he, but her core of orphan's toughness, her wifely monopoly on domestic management, his softness of heart, his utter reliance on her for personal care, the totalness of his devotion to her—by virtue of all these considerations—I felt he could scarcely survive her by a day.

The image came to me of how athletic she had seemed on the tennis court the previous summer, when he had fallen, and of how ruddy she had looked on the occasions we had seen her since. She was in Pittsfield's hospital, the Berkshire Medical Center, and I imagined her lying in a bed looking small and alone under the sheet and having somehow to confront the sickness within her. My father I pictured with his eyes swollen in bafflement and grief. The room rocked.

The news seemed too grave for the telephone, which is to me a business instrument, but I was bursting and called Barbara at home. She was fixing the children's dinner, at the most harassed domestic hour of the day. "Bad news from Pittsfield," I think I said. The kids were howling. "Mom's very sick. Cancer of the liver."

Barbara responded with a rush of feeling such as makes a man know in his bones that he has married well. "Oh, Steve," she said. She and my mother, to my deep delight, had always been full of uncluttered affection and admiration for each other. I could hear her crying. "Oh, honey."

It was incongruous. She was in the kitchen at home, I in my office twelve miles away, and yet we shared a moment of memorable intimacy. Strong emotion is a stimulant. It sharpens the senses and makes one aware of currents that ordinarily pass one by.

I went down the *Post*'s editorial alley to tell my editor I'd be going up to Pittsfield for a few days. It was too much. He came back into my office and shut the door. I'd always engaged him on a level of close but detached camaraderie. Now he flashed a gratifying openness to deeper feeling. We shook hands and I prepared to leave. The second of my editors walked up and took in the scene at a glance. I thought: I should tell her. She had twice recently been bereaved by family deaths. But, coat on, I simply nodded. She nodded.

It was towards deadline time and the newsroom was clattering. I went out on the street under a dark sky. Rush hour, with the cars going one way and faster on Fifteenth Street, had raised the traffic's pitch several tones. No one on the street, I realized, had any conception of what was going on in my head. Frowning at the prospect of the relative slowness and the company of strangers of my usual bus commute, I caught a cab.

Barbara came to me at the door. She offered words. I thanked her. It was a quick, complex exchange woven of different strands of love. Something she had said to the children had tamed their customary evening abandon and they presented themselves quietly for a kiss. We are in that sense a physical family, as my parents' family was. For years my father woke up his four children with a back rub, as now I wake up my four children—with a furtive pleasure, as they grow past the age of easy hugging, in finding a ruse to touch them.

I murmured to Barbara that I wanted to tell the children just what the situation with Grandma was. We had not previously made an occasion to discuss how we wished to play this end game with them. But once the situation was upon us, we both felt instinctively that a time of authentic family-making had arrived. We needed the children's support. We wanted them to take part in the family ceremony. It never occurred to us to spare them sad news or to try to preserve in their minds only the memory of happy and healthy grandparents. It was not even necessary for us to spell this out at the moment. We simply proceeded, reviewed it later, and never regretted it.

"Children, sit down," I said. We were in the television room off the kitchen. Just the overhead light was on, a harsh one to be on by itself, but I let it stay that way rather than set a stage. The four of them were primed for an important event.

"My mother is very sick with something called cancer and she is going to die. Not right away—you'll see her some more—but I don't think it'll be a long time." I went on a bit, but that was about the way it came out.

They were still. Becky, then nine, always quick and open in emotion, put her head down and sobbed, and went to Barbara. Dave, ten, more self-protecting, clasped his hands between his knees, hunched his shoulders, sniffed. Jimmy and Mike, six, looked small and bewildered on the couch. They twisted, each differently—fraternal twins.

The expressiveness and typicality of their reactions overwhelmed me. I did not want them to suffer or strike poses but I was gratified at this evidence of their love of their grandmother. I felt pride in having children capable of responding to a family imperative.

"What's cancer?"

"Something that decays you inside," I said. On a previous summer's hike with me up the mountain behind my parents' home, they had examined decaying leaves and the concept had stuck.

"When she will die?"

I almost had to laugh at the good journalistic quality of the questions, even as I observed that my amused reaction to the question had nothing to do with sorrow and mourning. "I hope not soon, but sometime," I answered. We all sat still, Barbara and I absorbing the children's concentration for several slowly ticking minutes.

Later she and I had a drink and sat long at table. I felt some need to start addressing the new family prospect formally, to make some clear personal statement of my mother's meaning to me and of the new family architecture her death would create. Yet then and at subsequent moments when I felt the same impulse, I was unable to put my mind into the gear necessary to move such thoughts forward. In a fairly short time I was to decide that it was not only too hard but unnecessary to perform that kind of mental exercise. I came to put trust in thoughts that arrived in my head under their own power. These considerations were authentic; these were reliable guides to feeling and acting.

And so, sitting at the table, Barbara and I spoke of particulars. We ransacked our memories for evidence of my mother's prior sickness or vulnerability. Some months back she had had some small rectal problem for which she had seen a doctor in New York. Since she had not entered a hospital, and since we had heard no more than that it was a "polyp," we had paid it scant heed. But we wondered now what it meant.

We thought of how incredible it was that someone of her truly legendary energy—she would run, heels clacking, to answer every phone ring, no matter how much the family scolded her for her compulsiveness—could be afflicted by cancer. We asked ourselves what "cancer" was, realizing, while nodding in dismay at my inadequate definition of it to the children, that nothing of what little we had picked up here or there equipped us to understand it now.

Most of all we pondered the likely impact of my mother's sickness and death on my father. The thought flashed through my mind that, with her gone, he would commit suicide—by crashing his car into a tree. He had never owned a gun and had once even related that he had hired a tentmate to clean his gun in World War I! It occurred to us that, to the extent that his own cancer could be affected by his attitude towards it, he would remove the internal chocks and let it roll.

How unfair was this reversal of death expectations at the end of his life, I thought. It had produced a situation in which a kind of weakness he had never had to face would rob him of the prospect of a mellow decline, dominate him, and spill over onto us. If "weakness" it was. I hesitated to judge.

Undressing for the night, I examined myself in the mirror. Healthy flesh, sick flesh, I thought. "Poor Mom."

Barbara, brushing her teeth, looked up. "I love you."

To bed.

THREE

Reversal

OUT THE SIDE WINDOW of the little deHavilland Twin
Otter flying up from JFK, my eye sought out the reas-
suring pattern of the mountains, roads, and individual
structures familiar on the Berkshire ground below. The
aircraft banked low in its final approach and I could see
our house, set off by the broad lawn in front and by
gently rising South Mountain behind. The plane slid
past the white slashes of ski trails at Bousquet's,
skimmed over the Wild Acres pond, and skidded to a
halt at the towerless terminal of the Pittsfield airport.

My father was there in the gray chill. He wore rubbers, his warm tan car coat and a wool-lined hat with pulldown ear flaps—the one my mother always chided him for wearing instead of the likes of the expensive Borsalinos he affected in other seasons. He bought these while on vacation in Europe, not through his own men's clothing store in Pittsfield: he enjoyed casing "the competition" on Bond Street and playing the boulevardier.

But he was no boulevardier now. His usually erect five-nine frame was slightly stooped. He looked thinner than the 170 pounds he had carried consistently, and with a certain puritanical pride in the implied self-discipline, since his youth. His long nose looked longer, his deep-set eyes more deeply set. "Stevie," he said, using the diminutive which, though it expressed to me a perverse unwillingness to grant my adulthood, I had become resigned long ago to let him use. We brushed cheeks in the traditional manner; his was unevenly shaven.

"Hi, Daddy," I said. "How's Mom?"

He said something I don't remember. His first words were a blur, not a report on his wife's condition but a barrier between the crushing implications of her sickness and his own total need for her survival. From a phone conversation with him the previous evening, I had learned nothing factual about her medical situation but had attributed the blank to the common family reticence to impart alarm at long distance. In it, too, perhaps was a hidden demand for the caller to present himself personally for the news. I accepted this. But now I wondered what I would learn on the scene.

We got in the car. He said she had spent a pretty good night; she was tired but the doctors said she could come home in not too long a time. The doctors, old and close family friends, were being remarkably attentive, dropping in continually to check, he continued. The nurses could not be more helpful and lovely—no request to them was ignored. This was the first occasion on which I noticed what became a recurrent theme. Not my mother's condition but the quality of her care, in particular the personal rather than the medical attention given her by doctors and nurses, was what preoccupied him, consciously at least.

Naturally I was happy to hear she was being well taken care of. But being generally short to a fault with people who do not make their points expeditiously and being genuinely concerned about my mother, I felt some irritation that my father did not impart the news. I looked carefully out the car window at the winter landscape and wished there were more snow.

Signboards at the hospital announced new-construction plans. Why must the patients pay to build the doctors' money-making factory? I asked myself, at once feeling uncharitable at assigning selfish motives to the very group of people who were tending so faithfully to my mother. We brushed through the lobby. It was crowded, disconcertingly so, with people waiting, watching television, munching machine snacks, or just standing around. The elevator was more comforting. Nurses chatted, discreetly avoiding matters that might impinge on the anxieties of visitors.

"Hello, Mr. Rosenfeld," a nurse said to my father.

He had lived in Pittsfield his whole life—very few Americans now live and die in their birthplaces, I thought—and rarely went anywhere without encountering people whom he knew, or who knew him. He bowed in his usual elaborate manner, as well as space permitted. "How's your mother?" he replied.

We stepped out into a muffled corridor and I followed him past the nurses' station to my mother's room. He paused at the door, hand on the corridor rail, leaned in, and beckoned me in.

My mother was in a bed (one of two in the room) near a window looking south toward our house. She seemed pale, and the usual contrast between her healthy complexion and nearly white hair was missing but otherwise only her eyes—careful, quiet—suggested that she was ill. She had not yet lost weight. Nothing one could take in immediately from her appearance or manner bore out the somber prognosis that had been relayed on the phone the previous afternoon.

Startled but gratified, I embraced her. Ordinarily she was brief and cheerful in showing affection to members of the family. Now she held my head down for a long silent minute. "You shouldn't have come," she said. "Did you have a good flight? How is Barbara? How are the children?" I swallowed at her determination to discharge her imperial grandmother's role. "Daddy," she said, "did you find Steve all right?"

He kissed her. They began speaking of what arrangements had been made for his meals during her hospitalization. Before marriage (at age thirty-six) he had lived with his married sister; after marriage he and my mother had had a live-in housekeeper, Eva Humphrey, for thirty years; and when Eva had retired back to the family farm my mother had cooked. So he had never learned much more in a kitchen than to boil water and he could not cook for himself.

It took some moments before I could start asking her how she felt. The gist of her reply was that she should soon be leaving the hospital. She held my hand and we spoke of many other things.

"Take Steve out to a good dinner," she ordered at the end of the afternoon. "Have a steak."

"It's a good thing you're able to give us your advice," my father countered. "We'd go hungry."

I was somewhat dazed to find them slipping back so swiftly into well-worn family ruts. My father and I headed for the Log Cabin on the Lenox road, one town south of Pittsfield, talking of my work, the stock market, what have you. It seemed somewhat unnatural that we should not be discussing family affairs but I was trying to pick up on what I felt were my father's wishes. Face to face at dinner, I figured, we would talk.

Yet entering the restaurant we bumped into an old

family friend, who was there alone, and when we discovered it was his seventy-seventh birthday, my father, with an effusive display of bonhomie, insisted that he join us. The double opportunity to show off a son and play the host swept him past a situation plainly configured for an intimate one-to-one.

Though he rarely drank, he ordered a glass of white wine and sipped half of it while I had a couple of martinis. The resultant glow was enough to give our odd bachelor party—one man's wife supposedly dying in a hospital, the second's divorced, the third's (mine) back home in Virginia—a semblance of gaiety. Steak was ordered. My father proposed a nice birthday toast. He indulged himself, as he sometimes did with my mother, by leaving a big tip, and I was inspired to take aside the restaurant owner, whom we knew, and tell him to expect both of my parents to come in for dinner soon, and to send me the bill. On the way out we met a woman whom my father introduced to me as an old high school girl friend. He was grinning. I had never heard even this trivial a disclosure of his romantic past (sixty-odd years ago!).

I remember this evening clearly. It was the last meal I know him to have enjoyed. It pleased me that I had made it possible for him.

By the next morning the mood had swung. My father began to moan. He said he had slept badly; he looked it. Motioning to his abdomen, he said he was in constant pain. We were at breakfast and his head dropped and he let his hands fall to his lap. A crumb, or some jam, stuck to his lip.

"My time has come," he heaved with a voice of great fatigue. "I never sleep at all. I am always in pain. The doctors can do nothing for me. I am of no value to anyone. I am only a burden to Beth."

Half of me filled with consternation at this (to me) unprecedented revelation of despair. The other half filled with dismay at the spectacle of what I took as his selfishness and self-pity in the face of my mother's greater trials. From what medical information was available at that morning moment, it seemed evident that my mother was—whatever her own attitude towards the process—dying. In the black shock of bringing her into the hospital earlier in the week, my father had told a friend he did not expect her to leave it alive. But here he was, fresh from last night's demonstration of vivacity and engagement with life, declaring that his professed distress merited family priority. I didn't know what to think. With no reasonable basis on which to make a comparative medical judgment, I shrank from contemplating the dizzying question of which parent was somehow worthier of the privilege, which is what it now seemed to be, of dying first.

My father sat there at the breakfast table and I sat there. "I'm sorry you feel so bad," I said lamely. He took my words as an encouragement to repeat his lament. Elated by my good son's role of the previous evening, I now felt entirely inadequate to his and my mother's perceived needs.

By the time we'd gotten to the hospital, my mother was sitting up in bed. "See," she boasted, "I'm getting better." My father was subdued. She offered a detailed account of the comings and goings of the various medical people in her room that morning. I could not help but notice that she was much more specific about the symptoms of her roommate, an older woman then sleeping, than about her own.

I had been trying to reach her surgeon, Ralph Zupanec. Seeing him go down the corridor, I shot out.

"Oh, yes, I've been looking for you," he said. I thought he might draw me into a quiet corner but he simply moved to one side of the bustling corridor.

My father hesitantly poked his head out of the door. His presence in the consultation would inhibit Dr. Zupanec, I figured, and that bothered me, but both of them had better claims than I to determine who should take part. It occurred to me that my father would profit, in the sense of getting a clearer view of his responsibilities to his dying wife, if he got the medical word straight from Dr. Zupanec.

I was also curious to see how the doctor would handle it. I had the notion then that the only issue of substance was whether and when and how the patient should be "told" of a terminal illness. I was willing to concede that telling was a complex issue for a doctor, touching the psychological and emotional aspects of his treatment of a patient, but I saw no similar complexities in regard to telling the family: the members should be told so that they could help the person dying. That there could be a situation where neither patient nor family could be told definitively because the doctor could not pin down definitively what to tell, had scarcely crossed my mind.

Zupanec, a slightly built, kind-looking man, did not so much deliver a report as weave loosely his several separate strands of concern for my mother on the one hand and my father on the other. I perceived his design even as I found it personally somewhat unsatisfying. Yes, there was "a growth," he said. He had removed what part of it he could from the colon. It was in the liver. Perhaps it would be elsewhere. There was no way of knowing precisely what would happen now. Sometimes these things could go a rather long time. Chemical therapy would be begun as soon as she could handle it.

He spoke on, simplifying the medical terms, recounting evenly the diverse aspects of my mother's situation, inspecting my father closely as he went along. The patient should be told of all of this, he concluded. He always thought it best.

My father nodded gravely from time to time, saying nothing and leaving it to me to carry the questioning. I caught his eye wandering off. "Thank you, Ralph," he finally said.

I said, "I appreciate your talking with us."

The doctor scooted off on his rounds and we rejoined my mother. "Such a nice man," she said. "What did he say?"

"He expects you to leave the hospital soon," my father answered.

Zupanec had not transmitted the hard-edged information I had wanted. His prognosis, though somewhat less dire than I had expected, was vague. He had held open a rather broad spectrum of uncertainties. He had not even clarified just what—and when and how—my mother would be told about her own troubles. But obviously he had said enough, or he had stated his prognosis in a way, to ease the anxieties—what they were I did not then fully understand—that were clouding my father's mind. My mother, too, seemed content.

I was disconcerted by the apparent disinterest of both parents in learning more about a matter of the deepest significance to them. My filial competence entitled, even obligated, me to take some sort of guiding role, I felt. At the same time, I had a countervailing sense of being the fourth person in the three-person crowd of parents and doctor. I could see no easy alternative to joining what amounted to the gentle conspiracy they had devised—one which plainly suited all the conspirators. Nor was I at all confident that a more direct and explicit approach would serve anyone's needs but my own. The more I pondered it, sitting in the hospital room, the more I thought that this was a poor time to expect a personality change, which was in effect what would have been required for either of them to take matters more forcefully into hand.

I had been in Pittsfield barely twenty-four hours, but I had accomplished my mission of seeing for myself what the situation was. I made plans to fly out on the regular flight to New York late in the afternoon. On this and on the dozen or more subsequent trips I would take to Pittsfield before both parents had died, I was similarly "mission-oriented." Once I had surveyed the scene or worked out whatever new arrangements needed an input from me, I grew impatient and—not without some mild guilt pangs—began to feel the call of family, work, tennis, even parties.

Not once did either parent ask me to linger or indicate any unhappiness that I was leaving too soon. On the contrary, they exercised to the end of their conscious days the same determination not to impose on their children's time that had made them such successful parents, to my mind, throughout my adult life. They would fly all the way to Washington for an annual visit, for instance, and despite our urging stay no more than two nights, sometimes only one, saying, "We don't want to overstay our welcome."

"Love to Barbara," my mother said from her bed. "Hug the children for me. Tell them I can't wait for them to come in the summer."

Just a day before, I had thought she was dying. Now it was not so much astounding as quite credible that she would be receiving her grandchildren in the coming August.

Only as my father drove me out to the airport, did the implications of this apparent change in my mother's fortunes sink in. Under the deadline pressure of the plane's departure schedule, he pressed forward a new line of conversation. He spoke earnestly and with the clarity of careful preparation. He was afraid, he said, of "leaving Mother alone." How would she take care of herself? She had been with him for so long. She hated spending even one night alone in their big and rather remote house. On one of the few occasions in their married life when he had been out of town alone, she had checked into a hotel—this was news to me. "You children" would of course do what you could but you had your own lives to lead in other places. It would be especially hard on Beth if she was alone and sick.

Clearly, in a complete turnabout from his earlier expectation of her certain decline, he had decided to read Zupanec's consultation and my mother's determinedly upbeat manner as evidence that she would survive, and survive him, after all. That meant to him that he could fulfill his plan and hope to die first. It was not death that he feared—we were to talk more of this in later months—but loneliness, living without his wife.

That much was evident to me in what he had said,

indirect as it was. His lifelong code and crust of manly self-reliance had not yet broken enough to permit him to say so more directly but I was moved that this man, who had never approached me in anything faintly close to this degree of intimacy, should approach me now. Yet it was evident, too, that he had something more on his mind. There was a palpable urgency. We were only minutes from the airport. It would not be an easy conversation to keep going once we had arrived and broken the seal of the car.

I remember a moment of recognition. It came to me that what he was really asking was my understanding, almost my permission, for him to die on his own original timetable—to die first. But to do this he needed the assurance that his widow would not have to pay an intolerably heavy price for what he seemed to acknowledge was an essentially selfish decision, one at odds with the solicitude he had always shown toward her.

I felt a circle closing. Such was my pity for him that I never thought to summon him to his putative responsibilities. Nor did it occur to me that their respective medical fates would be unfolding on a calendar affected only arguably, if at all, by their own conscious decisions. Instead, in words I have not regretted, I told him that it was characteristic of his affection and concern for her that he would be worrying about how she would fare alone. But he would be leaving her not just a house and the financial wherewithal to assure her comfort, but a loving family and devoted friends who would surely ensure her good care. "Plus, she is a very tough bird," I said. I meant it all, especially the last.

My father looked doubtful.

"You've provided her with everything so that she can get along without you," I threw in, a bit apprehensive even as I uttered the words that I might be going a step too far. "She won't need you."

My father, at the wheel, dipped his head in my direction. "Stevie, thank you," he said.

FOUR

Pittsfield

Pittsfield, city (1970 pop. 57,020), seat of Berkshire co., W Mass., between mountain ranges on branches of the Housatonic River; inc. as a town 1761, as a city 1889. The city is the metropolis of the Berkshire resort area. Electrical products are produced. Oliver Wendell Holmes lived nearby, and "Arrowhead" was Herman Melville's home from 1850 to 1863. —*New Columbia Encyclopedia,* 1975

IT WAS now that Pittsfield came into its own focus, not merely as the place where my parents were playing out their lives but as a party to the play. I was slow to recognize this life-sustaining, placentalike quality of the place. Popping up for quick weekends, even settling in for longer periods at vacation time, I had what was probably an exaggerated notion of my own importance to the two—later on to the one—of them. Indeed, when my father died, my sister Jayn and I both discussed with my mother whether she might wish to move in with one or the other of us rather than to be "alone in Pittsfield." Less ego than innocence was responsible for this misperception, I think. I simply did not have the imagination before the fact to see the part the town was to play.

I had left Pittsfield some twenty years before to take on the world. The city had become a place to which I returned principally, if not only, in pursuit of family pleasure. Barbara and I liked my parents immensely, we wanted our children to get a sense of generations and family heritage, and winter or summer it was a marvelous spot to go for vacation. What with the big house, the tennis court and swimming pool, the ski area scarcely a mile up the road, the woods in back, the household help who fixed the meals and cleaned up after the kids, the family friends who streamed up the long S drive to pay calls, the doting grandparents— what with all these things, "Pittsfield" meant to me mostly my parents' place on South Mountain Road.

"The Rosenfelds'," a lot of people called it. Our cousin Callie Wilson called it "173" (One Seventy-three), after the house number; years before, Jayn had painted the number and a G clef, emblem of my father's music, on the mailbox down on the road. On her stationery my mother had long used the designation "Twins Hill," bestowed when Eric and I were born in 1932—neither Rick nor I used it. Often I had reflected that when we came up to Pittsfield we could go for days without leaving our property.

I could but they couldn't. As much as my parents loved their South Mountain Road home, they were embedded in their community to a degree that I, shallowly rooted on my own in a metropolitan suburb which did not even exist until after World War II, needed the time of their dying to perceive.

My father's father Jacob, emigrating from Dettelbach, Bavaria, in 1866, as a boy of sixteen, had lived a typically marginal-period existence—apparently he was in the rag business—before stepping up to become a peddler in the Hudson River valley, and stepping up again to open the "Bon Ton" men's retail clothing store on Pittsfield's North Street in 1872, at about age twenty-two. In 1869 he and eighteen other "Israelites," thanking God "for the helping hand He extended to us in this strange land," had founded "Ansha Amonium" synagogue (as then spelled) in Pittsfield. An early photo of Jacob shows a short man with a dark mustache and a stern expression; age mellowed his visage.

He married Nina Levy of Albany in 1882; her widowed mother was of sufficient station to send out printed wedding invitations. Two of their daughters died in infancy. Of the four children who survived, the oldest, Zeno, ran away from home as a teen-ager and, notwithstanding an unverified report that he was seen working on the Panama Canal, was evidently never heard from again. My father, considering Zeno's flight or expulsion, whatever it was, a family scandal, invariably evaded our occasional questions about him. There was another brother, Stanley, who went into the family store, and a sister, Ruby, who married a doctor and also stayed in Pittsfield. Jay, the youngest, was born in 1895. The family lived at a house (since gone) at 196 Francis Avenue, then as now a working-class neighborhood. As much German as English was spoken in the home.

My father seems to have made only one serious effort to leave Pittsfield. Recognized as a hometown musical prodigy upon finishing high school in 1912, he sailed for Brussels to study violin. His European stay was underwritten essentially by his brother Stanley, who had been pulled out of high school a few years earlier—at their father's first stroke—in order to sustain the family business. Stanley was dutiful but "heartbroken" to leave school, my father wrote in an unexpectedly confessional newspaper ad (one in a long series of institutional "Rosenfeld Reports") published on Stan's death in 1961. I often wondered if Stan's family-defying marriage to a Catholic was in part his response to the heavy demands of family discipline—the same demands that had driven Zeno to Panama or beyond.

All his life, in files I discovered after his death, my father kept the little black notebooks in which he had recorded every centime ("carfare—10" "pastry—15") of his twenty-month Brussels sojourn. I sent those notebooks on to my brother Peter, a professional musician who had studied cello in Paris for the year after his own high school graduation. With the outbreak of World War I, my father departed Europe, continuing his musical studies in New York.

On March 25, 1916—again, in a letter I did not see until his death—his sister Ruby wrote from Pittsfield: "Dad was taken sick yesterday. . . . Stanley needs you. . . . Pack up all your belongings . . . as if you were coming for good." In detail, Ruby instructed him to make the stricken Jacob believe, in his weekly letter home, that his musical son was merely coming on a routine spring vacation for a brief stint in the store. No Zeno, Jay complied.

The last appeal my father received to rejoin the family—a gratuitous one, under the circumstances—came while he was serving in the American Expeditionary Force in France in 1918; these complete the family letters he saved in his files. "With God's help return to your folks sound and well," his father wrote in the painfully crude scrawl of a right-handed person forced by stroke to use his left hand. "When I think of what a fine penman he was, I am much effected," added his mother in the same letter. "Return to us."

I was to hear from my father much the same prayerful appeals when I went off in 1953 to what we all figured would be combat in the Korean War; three weeks later the truce was signed.

My father, who had Jacob's elaborate prestroke penmanship, applied for a commission in intelligence while still in France. Former U.S. Senator W. Murray Crane, Berkshire's ranking aristocrat, recommended him. He was rejected, the retained documentation shows, because his father was German-born. He had made a sentimental journey to Dettelbach, his father's birthplace, during his student days in Brussels. He was not to return to Dettelbach for another sixty years, taking lunch then with his wife in the inn in which he had spent the night in 1913. Mustered out of the army in 1919, he came back to Pittsfield for good.

I have always thought that the accidents which kept my father in Pittsfield were boons in disguise. I pressed him on the point several times and he conceded as much. The family business prospered, making him more comfortable than any conceivable musical career could have done and putting him in an excellent position to follow music as an avocation and to pursue other interests as well—travel, community uplift, Jewish causes, the education of his four children in paths leading away from Rosenfeld's Men's Shop and Pittsfield.

It was more than a matter of money. Owning a good business in a growing town at a growing time in America allowed a Jewish merchant of modest origins to become a certain figure, a kind of proprietor of the community. Liberal in social impulse, conservative in economic impulse, my father epitomized and espoused the ideal of the locally rooted and tied independent entrepreneur committed to community service as well as profit.

"It will be a sorry day for this city and for all American cities if and when business is conducted by absentee owners to whom the community is only something to slip under the microscopes of the Madison Avenue researchers, and when there will be no one sensitive to the needs of the city such as the Englands have been for a wonderful century," he wrote in open tribute to another Pittsfield merchant family, and in disguised tribute to his own, in 1959. He was pleased to be a Rotarian for half a century.

Growing up, I often had occasion to bask in the deference accorded "one of Jay Rosenfeld's boys" or "a Rosenfeld." Even many years later, when Barbara and I rented a cottage on Stockbridge Bowl in my parents' last summer, the agent, Claude Parker, informed us that he had now done business with "three generations of Rosenfelds"—he had been taken by his father to buy his first suit from Jacob.

Again that summer something happened to make me

think that, for a long period, purchase of a good suit represented for many people a memorable initiation into the middle class: thus did a merchant play the role, itself status-laden, of conferring a higher status on others.

I dropped into Samale's Pharmacy on Fenn Street, built on a corner that had earlier been occupied by Temple Anshe Amunim, to pick up some pills. "One of Jay's boys?" asked Giro Samale behind the counter. "How's your father? I met him when I came over from Italy in 1921. I was eight years old, wearing short pants in the snow, and my father brought my two brothers and me into Rosenfeld's for a suit and coat. We paid five dollars every Saturday."

My father rarely brought business home from the office. We children played guessing games based on his detailed knowledge of customers' suit sizes. He relished the story (apocryphal?) of an encounter with a customer who stopped him on the street to complain his trousers didn't fit. Irritated thus to be importuned, my father had him turn around, hike up his coat, and bend over; and then he walked away. He had no regrets that none of his children followed him into the store.

Then, too, by chance Pittsfield became perhaps the premier musical city, outside a metropolis, in the country. In 1918, Elizabeth Sprague Coolidge established a summer music colony on South Mountain, the same mountain on which my father later built his house. There she began the projects which made her the century's principal patron of chamber music. Returning from "my war," my father became a Coolidge protégé and thus assured himself lifelong association with musicians. At exactly that time, Marjorie Miller, arts-minded daughter of the local newspaper publisher, recruited him to write music reviews for the *Berkshire Eagle*. He did reviews for fifty-five years. In the 1930s the Boston Symphony Orchestra opened what became its regular summer concerts and school at Tanglewood in nearby Lenox. Meanwhile, my father promoted or led local amateur performances of good music.

Music filled our home. We boys carried the arthritic Mrs. Coolidge, a hefty five feet eleven, up the stone front steps in a sling chair to hear chamber music sessions at which the likes of Budapest Quartet members played with my father. The names and the non-name professionals from Tanglewood trooped in, often for tennis as well as music. All four of us children were steered early into music lessons; with two, it took seriously. Arpeggios were always being dashed off on the piano when somebody walked by. The late-night clacking of a typewriter signaled that somewhere in Berkshire County a public concert had been played.

In August, 1974, after my father had gone through his first cancer siege, he on the viola, Peter on the cello, Jayn on the flute, and Sheldon Rottenberg of the Boston Symphony on the violin, played a chamber music concert in the South Mountain hall. "Family affair at South

Mountain," the *Eagle*'s headline on the substitute critic's (favorable!) review read. A post-concert photograph of the three musical Rosenfelds took front and center position among the several dozen family photos on the piano. Peter and Jayn played again at South Mountain, in a concert mounted as a memorial, the summer after both parents died.

My mother, before coming to Pittsfield, had never had a permanent home or family core to which she might have been drawn back. She kept no files, physical or mental, and did not indulge even the mild bittersweet nostalgia in which my father coated his past. The only manifest acknowledgement of her origins was the classic wedding photograph of her parents which she kept in the bedroom. Her father, Samuel Kaufman, a very tall man, sits stiff and proud, top hat in lap, in a high-backed wooden chair. Her mother, Rose Axelrod Kaufman, in heavy flowing lace, stands in haunting serenity, hand on his shoulder.

Samuel, a mathematics teacher, had fled Russian Lithuania to avoid army service in the Russo-Japanese war. Settled in New York, he sent for his wife and three daughters, of whom two, Elizabeth and her identical twin Frances, had been born just before his departure; Mirian was four years older. He gave his daughters math problems at dinnertime, conditioning dessert on the answers, Francie later recalled.

Orphaned at about age eight, my mother was self-supporting at age fifteen or sixteen, and a prize-winning speed typist—she always typed like a fury. Her employers were Henrietta Szold and Rabbi Stephen Wise (my namesake), both leaders in the American Zionist movement. At age twenty she was national executive secretary of Junior Hadassah. In 1931 she was a worldly-wise twenty-five-year-old who danced at the Apollo and hung out with Christopher Morley's set. She and her twin had met the writer on the *Caronia* returning from Europe when, by family telling, he saw them playing deck tennis and decided that the backs of their heads looked like Joseph Conrad's. Although she had already seen *Green Pastures*, she agreed to go again with a blind date from Pittsfield. Three months later, on June 14, 1931, she and my father were married.

In Pittsfield she applied her formidable energies, and what I gather was a powerful pent-up nesting instinct, to family and community. Despite coming near death of peritonitis in the Caesarian delivery of Eric and me on July 26, 1932, she had two more children, Peter, born May 14, 1936, and Jayn, November 10, 1938. When her children went their own separate ways, without breaking community stride she took a paid job as director of patient activities at the Austen Riggs Center, a mental hospital down-county in Stockbridge. An *Eagle* article telling of an award given her in 1961 toted up her terms of service to various civic organizations and identified her as "Lady Who's Done Good for 134 Years."

My father retired and sold his store in 1963 at age sixty-eight. My mother retired from Riggs to be at home with him. As did he, she stayed involved with many other interests—in her case, tutoring, serving on a board or two, beginning Italian, playing tennis and skiing, traveling to Europe every May or September (they picked those months because they wanted outdoor walking weather but not at the expense of Berkshire summers), seeing friends, still running hard.

My parents were very fortunate people, and not merely because of their qualities, which were considerable, and the undoubted good luck of their lives. They lived long in one place—my father for virtually all of his eighty years, my mother for the last forty-five of her seventy. They invested themselves heavily there. Much of the fundamental tranquillity with which they both approached death, I believe, arose out of their true and certain knowledge that they had made a wise investment in Pittsfield. Little matter that they had made it out of contrary psychological compass settings, my father in fulfillment of a rather authoritarian family's demanding tradition, my mother in quest of a tradition that her own disintegrated family had never been there to demand: two characteristic immigrant-family strains.

Pittsfield was more than a lovely place, more than "the metropolis of the Berkshire resort area" and a city where "electrical products are produced," to cite the *New Columbia Encyclopedia*. For my parents, in their time, it had a notable character of its own: in its individually comprehensible size, its easy access to New York and Boston, its fairly stable pattern of community institutions and commercial traditions, its hospitality to cultural and religious diversity, its openness to the upwardly mobile. Unquestionably their lives would have been very different, probably poorer, if they had lived almost anywhere else.

They gave a great deal to Pittsfield. They got a great deal back. I refer not just to status and recognition but to the opportunity to pursue self-fulfillment, and to offer service, in a framework in which individual people and the community in which they live can match up face to face. Most of us, living in larger and stranger and more disjointed places, never know the particular satisfactions of the kind of integrated unalienated personal-civic life style that my parents experienced and exemplified in Pittsfield. So it was that the South Congregational Church put on a memorial performance of Ernest Bloch's *Sacred Service*, the Sabbath liturgy of the Jewish service, when they died.

A generation of American writers savaged the ways and values of small-town business America. A succeeding generation of American Jewish writers projected their own revolt of the sons against a similar milieu. I read their novels and was influenced by them and by the currents they portrayed but, through observing the actual histories of my parents, I arrived in time at a more accepting judgment. In the light of what is now perhaps the consensus critique of postindustrial urban American society, the Pittsfields turn out to be not such provincial and tortured places after all.

"You had to leave Pittsfield to learn so much?" my father said sarcastically to me in a particularly terse moment in my late teens. I forget what the argument was about but I remember his defensiveness about the town.

"When you got married, did you think you were coming up from the big city to the sticks?" I asked my mother in our last extended conversation before cancer smothered her speech.

"Oh, yes," she said, "but Pittsfield was good to us."

There the custom continues of allowing every deceased person's funeral caravan to roll slowly down the main street, through the red lights, on the way from the houses of worship at one end of town to the Pittsfield Cemetery at the other.

At a certain point in the sequence of dying, of course, a community or city, however securely banked in one's bones, reduces itself to the handful of people who gather by the side of one's bed. This is the ultimate occasion for receiving back a lifetime's investment in friendship and love. Both my parents received a breathtaking quality of devotion from their friends. Finally this was what "Pittsfield" meant to me.

FIVE

Slowing

THE PROSTATE, which surrounds the male urethra, is an organ associated with sexual function. It is, as medical writer Gilbert Cant has put it, the gland where the bulkiest of the three ingredients of sperm is manufactured and where all are blended for export. Prostate disorders are among the commonest afflictions of the modern American male, found among sixty percent of those over sixty years of age and among ninety-five percent of those over eighty. Cancer of the prostate is the severest form of prostatic disorder, constituting the third-ranking cause of cancer deaths among men.

"Cancer is the ogre," according to Cant, "because of dif-
ficulties in early detection and because, once it starts to
spread, it tends to spread widely through much of the
body."

So my father was, in a certain medical sense, merely
the typical American male. He was seventy-eight and a
paragon of good health when his sickness struck in London in May of 1974. It was cancer of the prostate and it
was not detected early. The bone scan ordered up by
his regular doctor, self-described "primary physician"
Herbert Glodt, revealed that the cancer was already
"extensive," having spread to the lumbar vertebrae and
to the ribs on the right side. This was the explanation of
the London hip pains.

Herb Glodt told my father that his condition was
serious but that of all malignancies, this type was the
one most amenable to therapy. My father received the
news gravely but calmly. At once, Dr. Christopher Mamonas, a urologist who had taken over the practice of
my father's late brother-in-law, performed a "TUR," a
transurethral resection, removing twenty-seven grams
of swollen cancerous tissue. Therapy of female hormones, which can inhibit cancer of the prostate, was
begun. An orchiectomy, removal of the testicles, was
advised on the theory that male hormones promote
cancer of the prostate. This my father resisted. In a few
days, his general condition was "satisfactory," though,
Dr. Mamonas reported at the time, "He is somewhat

depressed at the thought of having to have carcinoma and of potential bilateral orchiectomy. In any event, his condition has stabilized and he is discharged at this time."

He went home to his wife, herself then still full of health and vigor; to music and tennis; to his newspaper work—reviews of all the Tanglewood concerts that summer plus his regular weekly *Eagle* column of music and musing called "As I Hear It"; to his tray lunches on the terrace, where he would snooze after eating with the morning's *New York Times* rumpled on his lap. Religiously in the afternoon, he retreated to his bedroom, closed the door against the grandchildren, and napped. While swimming he wore an undershirt to cover the slight breast development that had resulted, despite cobalt therapy, from the female hormone treatment. Otherwise he made few concessions to his sickness. He looked hale and pink.

But the cancer was quietly spreading. In the fall, as the enlarged seasonal family presence on South Mountain Road dwindled to the normal complement of two, as the maple and beech behind the house were bared, my father's beat slowed. He ached and complained of the cold, moving his locus of daily routine early from the unheated sunporch to the snug "new room," a den which had been built as part of an addition about 1938.

Late in September, the new element of my mother's illness forcefully intruded. Abdominal cramps and some rectal bleeding had required her to undergo a series of tests in Pittsfield and then a particularly exhausting colon examination in New York. She had lost consciousness in the car as my father picked her up at the specialist's East Side office, and because it was raining and dark and the rush hour and because of his own near panic, he felt he could not stop to seek help. One hand on the wheel, the other on his wife, he had driven in desperation until he was out of the city and until she had returned to awareness. It was to him a savagely depressing foretaste of what was to come, and when I heard about it later I cringed.

Meanwhile, Dr. Mamonas was receiving both him and my mother outside of office hours in Saturday morning sessions set up to afford them special tranquillity. Softly, he advised that the long-delayed orchiectomy was becoming unavoidable in order to remove the main source of the male hormones thought to be spreading the cancer. My father saw and feared the operation, Dr. Mamonas later told me, as depriving him of the last identifying badge of his manhood and as terminating the capacity for general activity which was central to his self-image. I suspect further he saw it as symbolically ending his role as his wife's protector.

He went home from the hospital the day after the operation in December feeling fine. But the next day, Mamonas reported, he fell apart: "You just say, 'Oh, what the hell, this is the end.' " Male hormones contribute a sense of well-being; people in their fifties who are depressed are sometimes treated with these hormones to make them feel better. This is what my father, at a time of crumbling anyway, had now lost. And although—fortunately—he did not know it, he had lost it for nothing. His cancer turned out to be of a sort not pushed along by male hormones after all.

I went up to Pittsfield in January and was shocked at his weakening, the more so that at the time I was not aware of the immediate triggering cause. My father's face looked slack. Embarrassment tinged the appreciation in his eyes at my arrival. To the usual portfolio of grandchildren's drawings and greetings that I had brought along, he gave only a passing glance. He was strong enough to carry an armful of wood up from the garage to the "new room" fireplace, over my protests, but he then sank to the couch, flopped his head on my mother's lap, and sobbed. His body shook with an abandon that made me ask myself in some anger why he did not impose some self-control. He had always sneezed with that same sort of abandon: at the familiar anticipatory inhale, I had always frozen waiting for the convulsive relief. Now that was his common mode.

"I can't help it," he groaned. He talked of how fortunate he had been to marry "Beth," of how his love for her had grown in recent months even beyond the expectations nourished by a long and happy marriage, of how sorry he was to dump the burden of himself upon her.

She stroked his brow and blotted his tears, kissing the bald top of his head. "Now Jay," she said, "now Jay." She called him "darling," a term I'd never heard her use.

The winter sun set early over the house, situated as it was on the north slope of South Mountain. My father fell to recollecting some of the more easily quantifiable aspects of his life, rather as a businessman, which of course he was, draws the bottom line. He tallied the years of tuition (thirty-two) he'd provided his four children in preparatory school, college and graduate training, the trips (twenty-eight) he and my mother had taken to Europe, and the summers (fifty-five) he had written music criticism for the *Berkshire Eagle*. He stated that he had made it his practice to contribute more to the United Jewish Appeal for Israel every year than he spent on his own vacations. He had never totaled his income or assets for us children. I found these newly offered statistical measures considerably more meaningful. The tears stopped.

On the advice of several friends, I had recently read Elisabeth Kubler-Ross's *On Death and Dying*. Particularly valuable to me were its insights into the changing attitudes of the dying towards the process of their own death, and its counsel to the living to provide not just verbal understanding but "the silence that goes beyond words."

In the new room that afternoon and on many subsequent occasions, I found that just sitting there, listening attentively, shifting in the chair very little if at all, letting my father proceed at his own pace, countenancing long periods of silence—that this created an almost palpable calm that was as intense a form of communication as an animated conversation might have been in other circumstances. The hum of the clock in the FM radio became the dominant sound in the room.

As a journalist whose work is words, I could chuckle at the irony of inarticulate communication. It was much more appropriate, I thought, to music. I could recall the way my father held his bow still on the string of his violin until the last note's overtones had faded away. Regularly in his reviews he had criticized concert audiences for beginning their applause or getaway before the rests in the last measure had been counted to the end.

My mother drew me into the kitchen while she was making tea and, in a tone verging on the desperate, asked if I could talk to my father and do something about his depression. "He's not really as sick as he sounds," she said. She left us alone.

Again he went down his dark path, weeping, pointing to the pathetic spectacle of himself, saying that his life was pointless now. He had had seventy-eight good years, he said, but he wished to die. His face took on what was by now a characteristic scowl of hurt, anger, and self-pity. Plainly, he was aware at once of the physical and to some extent psychological disintegration taking place and of his diminishing capacity to handle the change. The one aggravated the other. I felt depressed and inadequate myself.

Barbara and I had recently completed a "Parent Effectiveness Training" course to see if we couldn't smooth out some family rough spots. P.E.T.'s overall contribution to family life turned out to be pretty transitory but it did yield a technique that I now tried to apply to my father. That was "active listening," a word or nod or grunt calculated to keep alive the flow of the speaker's feelings. As partial compensation for our previous failure to develop a habit of personal communication, it worked well enough for me to set aside my worry about its being somewhat too manipulative. For short spells, anyway, he could regain access to the shrinking enclosure of his old self-sufficiency.

I felt nonetheless that I simply could not provide the kinds of deeper assurances my father needed. I was in over my head. I told him so in just about those words and suggested he speak to his doctors.

He already had but he promised to do so again and asked me to call one of them, Herb Glodt.

I shook my head, knowing that I would be returning to Washington the next day and leaving my mother to carry the load of this weepy man.

Herb Glodt, making a "medical friendship" type of visit on his own time, had been dropping in every week or so. He was a sounding board for my father's marauding anxieties and he tried to raise his spirits at least to the level of his medical prospects, which were not yet all that grim. Herb's view was that the prognosis still merited the encouragement of hope rather than resignation. A deliberate and attentive man not put off—as I sometimes was—by my father's discursive conversational style, Herb sat with him for hours. They talked of cancer and life and many other things and at moments Herb wondered whether he was treating my father, a depressed cancer patient, or himself, a saddened friend. I could only be grateful that my father—perhaps more to the point, my mother—had support of this kind.

Later that winter I began what I intended to be a series of Pittsfield visits in which one child would come along each time. I savored the idea of tightening a three-generational link while it was yet possible. By the perpetual family calculus, the first child chosen was Jimmy, then six. He seemed the right one: still soft with baby fat and responsive (when in good humor!) to adults, he was our most "huggy" boy and—despite my father's effort at impartiality—his grandfather's evident favorite.

On the plane up, Jim flowered, as each of our children tends to do when accorded one or both parents' undivided attention. I warned him he could not engage in the usual yelling and jumping and would have to be sure not to bug his grandfather, who looked healthy on the outside but actually was sick on the inside. Jim asked for chewing gum. I had a sentimental vision of Jim and his grandfather settling into a chair for a warm reading session, as in earlier days.

But once we were there, my father took only the briefest notice of him, and my mother, though openly cheered by his presence, was too intent on catering to her husband to do more than give him occasional words and squeezes. Jim, a trouper, took it all in stride. Television and ice cream were the answer. Putting him to bed in "Jaynie's room," I said I was sorry the grandparents hadn't been able to do more with him but they had sickness on their mind.

"I know, Dad," Jim replied.

I suppose he did know. It made me glad that in past years, when no one's sickness had entered that house, we had given our children ample chance to get to know their grandparents and the Pittsfield scene. Jim's trip, supposedly the first in a series, was in fact the last. The three others accepted our explanation without fuss.

For the children's school vacation at the beginning of April we all drove up to Pittsfield—a 410-mile one-way trek we ordinarily made only once a year, in summer. Fearing to swamp my mother, who had just come home from her own cancer operation, we stayed at the cottage on the place of Stefan and Laurie Lorant a few miles south in Lenox. They, like other close family friends, were always ready to fortify the Pittsfield presence.

The pyramiding of my mother's troubles atop my father's had set me to wondering for the first time whether the right medical decisions for them were being taken. Friends in Washington pointed out that big-city specialists and leading researchers were available, especially for my mother, whose cancer seemed to be the more complex. It struck me that perhaps I might be derelict in not doing some checking on my own. Could my father, whose native son's and businessman's loyalty to his community was practically an article of faith, be leaving some out-of-town stone unturned? Had the previous September's nightmare trip home from the New York specialist spoiled forever his inclination to seek help beyond Pittsfield?

Over a bourbon in front of his fire, I put the question to Stefan, an author of books on Lincoln and the presidency and a vigorously opinionated man. By all means, he boomed, take your mother to Boston, to the Massachusetts General Hospital. He offered up the record of his own medical peregrinations as proof of the quality of his advice. My confidence in Pittsfield was wobbling.

The next day I phoned my mother's cancer specialist, Dr. Jesse Spector. He was young and brand new to Pittsfield and I had not met him personally. I reached him, only after several attempts, from a pay phone booth in Lenox next to the winter-closed Curtis Hotel, where my father had played in a dining room trio as a young man. Barbara was shopping for a dress across the street, having been dispatched by my mother, as was the invariable custom on our Berkshire trips, to buy herself something "and be sure to charge it to me—what else should I save my money for?"

The booth was frigid. Packed snow kept the door from closing and the sounds of passing cars whipped in. Unsure how to phrase my concern, I told Dr. Spector that friends had suggested that I take my mother to Massachusetts General or to some other specialists' spot.

"Go right ahead," he responded briskly, "if you want to." He knew who the good people were if we needed any help on names. He felt he should add, he said, that he was familiar with what other specialists might advise and it would not be different from his own counsel. Nonetheless, he understood why families might wish to look outside the city.

I had to strain to hear him speak over the noise of the traffic. I would consult with the other Rosenfeld children, I said.

But already I knew I would not press the matter further. For what Spector had said had crystallized in my mind a judgment I was already on the way to forming on the basis of much longer exposure to the other Pittsfield doctors. As Bob Maislen, a pediatrician and family friend who was keeping a discreet counselor's eye on my parents, had summed it up for me in a hospital corridor chat, the medical choices were being made with a nice sense of all the factors involved. The one phone call to Spector was hardly an exhaustive scanning of the medical alternatives, but I had been hunting (I acknowledged to myself) not so much for another doctor as for a reason not to deliver my mother to strangers. The Pittsfield doctors, I reflected, combined professional competence with a measure of personal concern nowhere else available. In the absence of any flicker of interest on the part of either parent—and no such flicker was to emerge—I felt no pressure to go out of town. I also felt a certain relief at not having to alter the medical arrangements already put in place by my father. All this was firm in my mind by the time I stepped out of the phone booth.

In the car, I told Barbara. She agreed. And later another consideration came to me: the impulse to seek ever more expert doctors and clinics reflects, after a point, a denial mechanism well known to medical people as a certain stage in everyone's confrontation with death. Sticking with the "Pittsfield doctors" of one place or another indicates not dereliction of filial duty but passage through that stage.

Later that same week, I carelessly got our car stuck in a snowbank at the Lorants' cottage. I had taken the wheel from Barbara insisting that I was the superior winter driver. The family was, under the circumstances, surprisingly gentle. We phoned my father to come pick up the children while we looked for someone to pull us out.

In ten minutes we spied his car backing up the half-mile-long hill road, narrowed by winter to a single track. He knew there was no place there to turn around. He was leaning out the car door and weaving a bit but he made it all the way up. It was rather a virtuoso performance, in a sense his last. Pleased as punch, he surveyed the black dirt that my spinning rear wheel had kicked up, as though to say he shouldn't be counted out just yet.

"Nice going, Dad," I said.

He took the children and we found a tow.

Such triumph, however, was fleeting. Practically his first words on my next trip were, had I read of the Van Dusens? Dr. Henry Van Dusen, the theologian, and his wife, being about eighty and sick, had together swallowed overdoses of sleeping pills. She died that day, he fifteen days later. A letter explained their act as a long-pondered decision taken for considerations of dignity. What did I think of them, my father wanted to know. His tone conveyed approval, almost envy, of what they had done.

I could not believe he could conceive of enlisting his wife—she was at the time, after all, apparently recovering from an operation, not sinking towards death—in a double suicide, however the idea might have appealed to him. Her spirit was too vital, too positive. Nor could I accept that, with the matter of his own death prior to my mother's settled as much as such a thing could be settled, he had a driving motivation to take his own life. The means would also pose a problem.

I felt, nonetheless, that he was looking towards circumstances that might yet arise—indeed, probably would—and that he wanted to start mustering the necessary rationale and self-mastery to afford himself the option at a later time. I did not shudder or veer away from the idea. The failing father of a close friend, first summoning the son in what he later realized was a bow of farewell, had retreated to the bathroom and shot himself with a gun from his collection—in order to cut short for the whole family the painfully ragged ending that otherwise surely lurked. My friend had portrayed the act to me as one of generosity and love, and I accepted it exactly in those terms.

I had also begun to think about the need and right of a dying person to manage his own fate—not just the terms of his care but the term of his life—rather than to surrender responsibility by default to others or to genuflect to a life principle that might or might not retain meaning as the end neared. Suicide as the break between a rich life and a harsh death seemed fitting enough to me—though inferior to the quick, clean death on a tennis court that had been my father's heart's desire.

So I said to him simply that I thought the Van Dusens had done what they honestly felt they had to do, that their decision was beyond anyone else's blame or praise, that each person had a right to think those questions out for himself. I paused and asked him what he thought about the Van Dusens.

No answer came.

I craved relief from the close, still house and went alone outside into the spring brightness on the mountain. Knowing from my last hike the previous summer that trees had fallen across the ski trail, I took an axe, though no one skied the trail anymore. A beech perhaps eight inches across at the base had fallen just below a little dip—a feature as clearly impressed on my memory, from dozens of climbs up and runs down as a boy, as a ski track in fresh snow. I heaved my back into the axe, feeling the force, listening for the thud and the echo, watching the cut taper nicely—I know how to use an axe. The severed trunk rolled off the splintered stump and I moved up for the next cut.

It was then I became aware that someone was standing quietly by. It was a friend, a lanky intelligent-looking neighbor who had been confined to home and neighborhood by a psychological condition for all of his almost forty years. We greeted each other. Philip inquired solicitously of my parents. He received with an understanding nod my report that I was clearing the ski trail. He knew the mountain from the kind of perennial season-round prowling that I'd had to abandon decades ago. With my brother, I had tapped the maples once, collecting buckets of sap. My mother boiled it down into a mere quart or so of syrup on the kitchen stove; she not only paid us for the syrup but had to repair the ceiling plaster loosened by the days of rising steam.

Philip had tapped the same trees for years, boiling the sap himself and also selling the syrup to my mother.

He was carrying the kind of radio receiver on which, he explained, he could pick up the Pittsfield police and fire calls from the top of the mountain. A click brought the staccato babble of municipal services to our remote slope.

I shied back.

Philip clicked off the set and, waving formally, moved on up the trail.

An odd encounter, I thought: we both were seeking clarity on the mountain. Turning back to the beech, I dug out a chip a good eight inches wide. I have it still.

SIX

Florida

SPRING CAME LATE to the Berkshires in 1975 and my father, always pridefully at ease with cold, worked up a harsh and almost personal rage against the delay. He could scarcely fault my mother for having had an operation in March which penned them in Pittsfield past the time when they otherwise would have planned a trip away. But he could and did grumble constantly about the place and the weather and his own malaise—all of a dark piece to him.

Had he erred by not selling the Pittsfield house and moving south years ago? he queried my mother, who took this heretical suggestion, like all similar ones, not as a question to be answered literally but as bile to be patiently drained away. She was an avid sun lover; the quip of a friend admiring her tan, "Are you that color all over?" had been set in the stone of family repetition. She herself was eager to escape the lingering Berkshire chill. What ultimately was holding them back, we Rosenfeld children realized from our floating watch on weekend visits and on the phone, was their need for someone to escort them to Florida and tend to them there. They were afraid to go alone. I went along.

Our plane to Fort Lauderdale, the Florida place they knew they liked, was to leave late Saturday afternoon from the Hartford airport, some sixty miles away. I got up to Pittsfield the night before and we went out to dinner with Karl and Marianne Lipsky, owners of an Americana business called Jenifer House down-county in Great Barrington, and faithful friends of all the Rosenfelds. When I'd worked for the *Berkshire Eagle* in its Great Barrington bureau twenty years earlier, I'd lived a while in the beautifully restored eighteenth-century Lipsky house in nearby New Marlboro. Karl brought drollness, Marianne sweetness, both a taste for style; and I was sure dinner with them would shift my parents fluidly into a holiday gear.

But the evening was a dud. We went to the Berghof, a new restaurant with a mountain view; my father barely noted it. The sight of our waitress, a pretty girl in a scoop-necked dirndl, ordinarily would have set him to observing, with a chaste twinkle, what a lovely young lady she was. Instead he asked her to turn down the Austrian background music. Revealing the layer of puritanical rigidity underneath his customary courtliness, he showed impatience at my ordering of a drink. Twice again the waitress was summoned to turn down the music. The last time, her politeness taut, she informed him the manager would not allow her to lower it further. Karl tried to pump in a little jollity but it didn't work. My mother was caught between returning the Lipskys' warmth and retreating for the sake of my father. I frowned to see for the first time that they could not savor the company of friends.

For a quick lunch the next day before driving to Hartford, we ducked into Samel's Deli on East Street. My father smiled stiffly to the owners, longtime acquaintances. My mother introduced me, and the usual Pittsfield knot—a review of the associations of Rosenfelds and Samels over the last sixty years—was neatly tied. We ordered and chatted idly.

Suddenly, without warning, my father leaped up from the table and ran to Dr. Herb Glodt, who was just entering with his wife. They exchanged words and Dr. Glodt led my father, crying and gesticulating, into a back office. Mary Glodt sat down for lunch with my mother and me. Personal relationships with the doctors' families continued and, for me, an out-of-towner, deepened during these assorted trials.

We guessed what had happened. My father, from

previous counseling sessions with Herb Glodt, simply could not let pass an opportunity to unload some more of his accumulated unhappiness. That he had broken down so instantly at the mere sight of Glodt gave me pause. But so what, if he created a semi-scene in a public place? I thought; if it made him feel better, fine. Anyway, these were no "public places" in Pittsfield. Samel's, smelling of hot Jewish meat and fresh bread, filled with people he knew, was familiar and easy. In a while my father and the doctor emerged. Everything seemed normal. We all had a coffee and left.

It was after 11 P.M. when my parents, limp from fatigue, and I arrived at the Sheraton Clipper Inn on Fort Lauderdale's ocean front. By some foul-up, the reserved rooms were gone. Their last bit of stuffing spilled out as the clerk's word struck. They sank onto a bench in the lobby. Horrified, I swept them and our bags into a new cab and, asking for the clerk's suggestion and telling him to phone ahead, shot up to the Bahia Mar a quarter mile north on the beach. Yes, the Bahia Mar—a marina-motel that figured in the Travis McGee thriller I happened to be reading on the plane—could take us in. The clerk there helped me park my parents in their room instantly. We had lost less than five minutes from the moment the Sheraton had shut the door.

Obviously it was great luck that a place as near and nice could put us up—we stayed there the rest of the week. But for days afterwards my parents shook their heads in wonderment at what they preferred to treat as my personal virtuosity in retrieving a disaster. "I don't see how you did it," my mother said. "Steve, you're wonderful." Luck aside, I had been quick and cool in a tight spot—a response they knew they could no longer muster. The emergency had produced warming proof to them that, as they declined, someone would be there. It was me in that instance, my sister and brothers in others.

The next morning I spent a tedious hour trying to find folding beach chairs that my parents could site and move about as they chose. The only ones available had to be used at an area half a mile up the beach. My failure turned my father to scowling about why had they come to Florida in the first place. I steered them towards the big elevated pool of the Bahia Mar—it was close to their room and had plenty of chairs, plus attendants.

White from winter, my father's frame looked frail and flaccid. The May sun began to redden him in patches that made him seem less healthy than ‹fevered. My mother dutifully oiled up, lay back as though to drown in sun, and browned. He spent hours, especially in the mornings, cataloguing his symptoms and interspersing feeble regrets at subjecting his listeners to the dismal recital. She put on lipstick and new dresses and peered at herself passing mirrors. We did not wander far from the inn. Sometimes we strolled along the dock where boats came in to take tourists out fishing, and inspected the trophies—big fish, looking sick and gray hanging head down out of water. To make sure that my mother, in her concern to take care of her husband, did not tire, I hung close by.

Barbara's arrival midway through the week cheered us all, especially me, and let my mother stop fretting that I was having no fun. To see Barbara linking her arm in my mother's or father's, drawing out a lively conversation, her dark hair bobbing, was a quiet joy. While they rested, we swam laps.

A stranger to Florida, I was seeing two of its special aspects—tourist Florida and old people's Florida: two separate spheres sharing a single-mindedness in pursuit of their respective goals and a detachment from what to me was the "real" life of the community. Given our own short leash, we observed our fellow tourists mostly at the restaurants, where rubbernecking and exhaustive menu study seemed to be the principal activities. Dinner was less an occasion for a good meal or a good time than an opportunity to see how one's appearance and manner compared to those of others. At Ratner's, a clattering Jewish place, menu and service had been tailored to turnover. Patricia Murphy's, trying hard, offered the anomaly of ostensibly intimate candlelight in a glass-walled room the size of a barn. From the Clipper, the view—east to the ocean, a mottled green turning to gray in the fading sunlight—dominated the table.

Actually, we liked most of these and other places. We ordered off the left side of the menu, as my father liked to say. In their case, dining had the purpose of therapy as well as pleasure. My father ate well enough but invariably complained later that he hadn't enjoyed it—an inconsistency we indulged. My mother ate as though she wanted to earn a battle star for each meal, and gained a pound a day. They had come to tourist Florida for rest and sun, nothing more, not for cure, not to drop out of the long march but better to gird themselves for it. They were there for a transient time and reason. They had no complaints.

Old people's Florida we saw chiefly in the visit we paid to my mother's older sister and her husband in their retirement condominium colony in North Miami Beach. We arrived for dinner on a mellow evening and at once heard from Miriam and Sam the kind of faintly defensive portrayal of life style that my parents, in their more natural and rooted circumstances in Pittsfield, would never have thought it necessary to make. Confirmed New Yorkers, Miriam and Sam had doubted that human life could be sustained outside of Manhattan. But the climate of Florida and especially the activity and supportiveness structured into their commune had won them over. I had half expected to find it ersatz but the place obviously was filling genuine needs of older people.

The quiet and manicure of the complex, inside and

out, however, indicated what was missing: children. Miriam begged for the latest photos of our four to add to the gallery which, I gathered, was a fixture of every apartment: evidence of the now-remote clans of which these old people, grouped here only with each other, had formerly been a contiguous part.

Presumably retirement communities are, for the people who choose to live in them, the best of all possible worlds. But different worlds are possible. I walked around the lawns with my uncle Sam, who had taken on for his wife as well as himself the burden of ascertaining the condition of my parents. I found myself feeling thankful that my parents had a community of their own, and a home of their own, to which to return to die. In them I detected no regrets about the world they had chosen for themselves.

Not since teen age had I spent so many consecutive and undistracted days with my parents. That time in Florida had a particular quality—deliberate, uncluttered, aseptic, though rendered somewhat brittle by our unspoken mutual awareness that we would take part in no similar passage again. Fort Lauderdale was the lull, all of us surely sensed, before the final storm—or whatever the final stage would be.

I wanted to do more than entertain or divert my parents. I wanted to convey to them a certain impression of what were the most important things in my life. I talked at length and rather guilelessly about my family and work, my likes and dislikes, my hopes and anxieties for the world, trying to go beyond the usual newsiness into the values that seemed to me at play. We say by the pool in the afternoon and dawdled over dessert at night.

My mother's eyes were sharp, her attention was sharp. My father might nap or gaze off or toy with a spoon but she listened and did not interrupt. I suppose I sounded like a lecturer. She never conveyed any reaction except that of affection and respect for my word and worth. She was a very level and accepting woman, and as a result of these and some further conversations, by the time she died I felt that I had said to her everything I wanted to say.

In fact, I had rather saved up a story, or a subject—music—for my father on this trip. A month or two earlier, we'd decided to give violin lessons to Jimmy, then six. He'd liked hearing one of his uncle Peter's daughters, even younger, play. Barbara scouted the neighborhood and was touted strongly on a teacher named Olga Gigante.

"Rosenfeld?" said Olga on the phone. "From Pittsfield?" As an underaged schoolgirl violinist, she had been slipped into the back stand of an adult community orchestra by my father, then its conductor. He later encouraged her to take the financial chance of entering music teaching as a career. Elated to be closing a circle, Olga jumped Jimmy to the head of her waiting list and started him out on a half-sized violin.

I told my father this story, with suitable embellishments, and then I told him that I'd begun playing the violin again myself after a full twenty-year hiatus in which some years the single time I'd picked it up was for a ten-minute demonstration before the children's nursery school class. Jim would saw away at his Suzuki songs. I'd play with him and keep going a bit when he stopped. Though I was not nearly enough of an instrumentalist to demonstrate the point, I was enough of a musician to know that the good sound comes from the right, bow hand and not from the left, fingering hand. At a point in each session, when I'd bumped up against the certain knowledge that I was years of practice distant from the sound my ear craved, I'd put the violin back in the case.

I'd also begun to listen again to violin records on the hi-fi. In the intervening years, the records of what I called "mature women"—Petula Clark, Barbra Streisand, Dionne Warwick—had monopolized our set. David Oistrakh playing the Beethoven concerto; Isaac Stern, an old acquaintance of my father's, doing the Bartok: they played not pretty music but the true tones, the sounds within sounds. They played, as my father had always put it, "in the string"—the way he had played.

My father received this accounting quietly. He had just decided, because of his failing strength, to dispose of his own violin, a lovely J. B. Guadagnini made in 1761. So responsive was it to the slightest physical command that in my hands, accustomed as they were to a far cruder, slower violin, it ran away the way I suspect a thoroughbred horse would repel a first-time rider's clumsy rein. I could imagine how much it pained my father to stop playing his fiddle—the violin was precisely what had transformed his whole life prospect. That was why I was offering him my kind of music recital: assurance that my part of the family valued what he had prized.

Yet, sitting by the Bahia Mar pool on that slow afternoon, I sensed I'd told him too late. The musical switch in him had flicked off. Nostalgia could not turn it back on even briefly. His love of music had narrowed to anxiety about how his violin would be treated in his estate.

What absorbed him considerably more than music was the question of who would care for my mother and him upon their return, he as an incipient invalid, to Pittsfield. He had fervently hoped that Carolyn Wilson, a niece without other family obligations who was working as a librarian in Connecticut, would move into the Pittsfield house and take over. Callie was a great favorite and, my father felt, he had been good to her. But Callie, though tugged hard by love and loyalty, felt she had to take advantage of an attractive study-job opportunity just then opening in Wisconsin.

She was, of course, entirely right. My father had the means to buy the necessary services and in fact he and my mother had already hired a perfectly marvelous cook, Alma Pinney. My mother's steady cleaning woman, Lorraine Hughes, and my mother herself could do what else was needed. My father, however, was thinking in terms of filling the principal family requirements with family members. I think he felt that, as the patriarch, he had a certain claim on Callie—in a way, more of a claim than he had on his own children, none of whom was in a position to return to Pittsfield for the duration. It vexed him that this one essential element of personal care seemed to be eluding his careful planning for old age. I sought to persuade him that everything would work out fine.

What with our attention centered on escort duty, Barbara and I had trouble settling into a vacation rhythm of our own. Evenings, after we'd deposited my parents early back in their room, were the only time we had for ourselves. One night we drove to Miami looking for the dog track but missed the turnoff and ended up muttering on the freeway. Another night we felt like seeing a movie but could find only *Shampoo*, which entirely fulfilled my low expectations for it and which was playing in a bizarre drive-in theater where seven other films were simultaneously being screened. On yet a third evening we were turned away from a recommended night spot for want of a reservation.

The morning of our departure, Barbara and I dashed out to the ocean for a last dip. "Not much of a vacation, honey," I said.

"With you it's always a vacation," she said back.

My parents' plane back to Hartford, where a friend was to pick them up, was scheduled to leave an hour or so after ours left for Washingtonn and we drove to the airport together. Quite ready to go, I welcomed the relief of having to tend by myself to the business of car and baggage. For a while I chatted with a waiting limousine driver. Rejoining our cluster, I was drawn aside by my father.

Glumly, wordlessly, he handed me a folded piece of cardboard cut from an old Rosenfeld's Men's Shop inventory form—he kept dozens of such pieces around for daily note-taking. It said, in his penciled script: "Meehan Funeral Home. No flowers. No eulogy—Peter has quotations. Cheapest possible casket. Cremation."

I felt suddenly tired and put upon. My father had a right to spell out the final details, but why did he have to lay it on this thick? This was not the way I wanted to be thanked for providing them a week in Fort Lauderdale.

My father was standing there forlornly, like an underpaid delivery man waiting for a receipt.

"OK, Dad," I said, "we'll do it your way. Have a good trip home."

SEVEN

August

IN JUNE, just before the 1975 Tanglewood season opened, my father announced to Pittsfield that he was dying. Hormonal therapy had proven ineffective, and he had just undergone a second operation to dig more cancerous tissue out of the prostate. Dr. Mamonas had found an uncontrollable "high-grade malignancy" and had had his associate inform me when I called that it would kill him within a few months. In his regular Saturday "As I Hear It" column, my father reported that after fifty-five years of music reviewing for the *Eagle*, "unreliable health reasons" were forcing a halt. He said he would continue recording "happy memories and reminiscences" in his weekly column. His headline for the piece was "Graduation."

It was a bittersweet term. The actual reviewing of concerts, I suspect, had never been what mattered most about newspapering to my father. His reviews—informative, knowledgeable, written in the prose of a self-educated man influenced by youthful reading of Gibbon and Macaulay, kind to a fault both to performers who did not meet his high standards and to composers who did not satisfy his mainstream tastes—were widely read. His and my mother's intermission and post-concert appearances in the left front corner of the Tanglewood Shed, to greet friends and chat with the musicians coming down off the stage, had become a familiar Berkshire social ritual akin to holding court.

But what he really loved was the opportunity his reviewing gave him to keep company with his friends at the paper. He loved shooting the breeze with all the journalists, young and old, in the newsroom; delivering his copy to Milt Bass ("Where's your crap, Jay?"); having a cup of coffee with the editor, Pete Miller, and the managing editor, Rex Fall. In retirement he had timed his daily run "upstreet" to the *Eagle*'s nine o'clock coffee break. At one point, growing older and fearing that Pete might be keeping him on for friendship's sake alone, he drafted a letter of resignation: I found it later in his files with a notation, "not sent on advice of EKR."

His various other activities outside the house he could

relinquish without much evident regret. The *Eagle* he clung to virtually beyond the end. I say "beyond the end" because in August, when pain and drugs stopped him even from doing his column, he had me, with Pete Miller's approval, pick out old columns to run again. The last photograph of him, taken without his knowing it by Stefan Lorant, a master at catching fact on film, shows him working on what was apparently his last piece. His eyes are sullen in the sockets, his mouth hard, but he is at his typewriter.

When my father came home from the hospital late in June, all residual family expectations of tolerably gentle death quickly dissolved. I went up to Pittsfield to see him. He could speak only of pain. He wanted no more operations, no more hospitals, he said, he wanted only for the doctors to ease the pain throbbing in his abdomen and shooting out beyond. At some hours he could read or stroll or receive visitors. At others he gasped and moaned.

On several occasions he asked if I could not instruct his doctors to give him a pill or an injection that would take him right out. He explained this request as a blessing for himself and as a salvation for his wife, who was by now receiving for her own cancer a kind of chemotherapy which produced pitiless nausea. It was unfair, he said, that she should have to care for him at a time when she was passing through such an ordeal of her own.

I did not broach his appeal directly to my mother.

But I did sound her out enough to conclude that she was numbed by his suffering and reconciled to his inevitable loss. Fortified by that conclusion, I phoned Dr. Richard Marcure—the associate of Dr. Mamonas, who himself was out of town.

Not knowing him, I found it hard to say what was on my mind but I told him that my father was having to abandon all the business and pleasure of his life, that he was overwhelmed by his own pain and by the burden he was placing on his wife, and that he wanted to die. If he had realized he was going to undergo another operation in his last hospital stay, I said, he would have said no. I had talked to my brothers and sister and thus could say that we children as well as my father were opposed to "heroic measures" to extend his life.

I finished up short, realizing that I had shied away from saying outright that my father wanted something to take his life away. Marcure responded guardedly, saying that he and Mamonas would consider all these things in their treatment. The conversation left me feeling dazed and dissatisfied, as though we were all— family and doctors alike—passengers on a ship with a stranger incommunicado at the helm.

By early August my father still occasionally felt well enough to want to drive, although the scars on the garage door and the scratches on the fenders of his Dodge attested to his loss of skill at the wheel. None of us, however, had the heart to insist that he surrender

this symbol and form of the active life. One afternoon
on the way to the Stockbridge Bowl cottage where my
sister Jayn and her family were staying for the first ten
days of August, he had a small collision at the tricky in-
tersection in the middle of Lenox. No one was hurt, but
all of us, hearing about it, stewed. Injury to himself or
his wife seemed a relatively trivial though gratuitous
risk compared to the cancers they already were facing,
but the possibility of injury to others was genuinely dis-
turbing. His deterioration soon mooted the question.
My mother had no further taste to drive herself.

Barbara and I had postponed for a year a long-
planned family ranch-and-river expedition to Colorado
in order to spend what we were sure was my father's
last summer in the Berkshires. With our children, we
replaced Jayn in the Stockbridge cottage on August 10.
Our plan was to drop by South Mountain Road daily
for tennis and swimming and perhaps lunch out on the
terrace.

The first week, the arrangement worked well enough.
We kept a buffer of time, space, or quiet between the
kids and my father. He scolded Becky, then ten, with
disproportionate asperity for breaking a folding wooden
"waterfall" toy he had bought in Europe years ago. "I've
had this fifty years and you broke it in one afternoon,"
he told her. Forewarned to expect erratic behaviour
from her grandfather, she held back the tears. Dave,
eleven, would carefully watch my father, taking in the

strangeness of his ways, and then turn back to his reading. The little boys played on or, depending, scrapped on almost as though he was not there. All four children would kiss him hello and goodbye every day according to family custom.

I wondered nervously whether any of them might make an uncomfortable point, in his presence, of his increasingly gaunt visage and slack manner. None did.

"Granddaddy looks old," Michael observed in the car returning to Stockbridge one afternoon.

"He is old," I said. "He's very sick. This summer is probably the last time you children will see him." We had kept the children well informed of the broad facts, if not the details, of their grandparents' condition. Their eyes now told them most of what more they needed to know. It seemed to me they understood the situation perfectly.

Because my mother was nervous about having to handle a crisis alone, either Barbara or I, with one child, settled into sleeping overnight in Pittsfield while the rest of the family went back to the lake. This usually meant that the six of us would eat not only lunch in Pittsfield but dinner, too. Alma Pinney, the Norwegian-born cook, could not have been more pleased. Fixing a meal for less than eight or ten ravenous field hands seemed to her a scandal. "Is that all you are having?" she would ask, with a faint smile, after we had demolished fare for a small brigade. Accustomed to a life style out of "Upstairs, Downstairs," Alma called me "the other Mr. Rosenfeld." Daily she brought fresh vegetables from her own kitchen garden ("They're not good if they're not fresh, you know") and her lemon pie was bliss.

But that was at the dining table. Day by day, practically in front of our eyes, pain ate into my father's consciousness like water filling up a sponge. The doctors' pills seemed no better than aspirin. He would subside briefly but then become wild-eyed. My mother's brow knit in deep dismay. He would retreat to his room and lie down and I would follow the two of them in there, quietly frantic myself but helpless to suppress the pain of cancer and the cancer of pain.

I asked myself what were the responsibilities of a son. And one Saturday afternoon I knew. Sitting downstairs in the sun porch, carrying on a dialogue with myself while the children played on the floor, I knew that if neither the doctors nor death came quickly to his comfort, then I would intervene.

The decision, which is what I felt it was, produced in me a buzzing and a calm: a measure of alarm, not so much at the personal risk, which I thought nominal, as at the audacity required to bring another's life to an end; and a larger measure of conviction that I would be fulfilling my father's will and doing the right thing. He had, as Jorge Luis Borges had put it, a "great hunger for death." The method I had in mind was smothering—slipping up to the room while he napped, leaning my weight and strength on a pillow, and then restoring the scene to normal. I did not think anyone else had to know, though I pondered telling a few family members in time. Our family discussions had produced a consensus tolerating, if not actively encouraging, such a course, I believed. And there was no one else there but me.

Looking back, I see that my plan may not have been so free of the risk of detection as I imagined, and my determination to carry it through might or might not have been sustained in the act. These are speculations. I am glad I was not tested. Because of circumstances I will shortly relate, the plan was never put into effect. It went into a closet of my mind.

I hauled it out, just for inspection purposes, only once thereafter. My father had died. Barbara and I went out for dinner in Washington and met a psychiatrist visiting from a distant state. He and I struck up a rapport and over after-dinner drinks fell into the kind of intimate discussion that, as Russians say, can be held only by two strangers meeting for the first and last time on a train. He had his own story to tell about the death of his own parents. I told him my story. He projected great understanding of the act I had contemplated. Whether it was the meeting "on a train," or the drinks and the late hour, or a psychiatrist treating (gratis!) a random patient, was and is immaterial. I had been profoundly reassured.

In any event, having assembled my plan on a Saturday, I awoke the next morning to find that my mother had been up for hours trying to beat down my father's pain. Throughout the whole period of his decline she tended him with a melting selflessness. On this morning in particular she seemed stretched to the limits of her self-control. We called Dr. Marcure for consultation and, towards noon, called him again to ask him to come. The Pittsfield doctors made scores of house calls to my parents during their travail. He was there in half an hour.

Stern and businesslike, he quickly verified what had been obvious even to me. The urinary tract was clogged by the growth of cancerous tissue to the extent that nothing could any longer pass through the catheter, emptying into a leg bag, that my father had been required to carry for some time. Marcure dismissed my mother and ordered me to assist him in trying to pump the urinary tract out.

It was for me strong stuff: a helpless, spread-eagled man writhing under natural pain so great that it all but blotted out the considerable additional discomfort (and indignity) of the pumping procedure. I thought to myself that this was my father's ultimate vulnerability, and if he could hold on, then I could do what I had to do. Marcure finished and told me to clean my father up and take him to the hospital for further relief.

I dressed him. His limbs were like rags. Incontinent,

he soiled his underclothes, once, then twice. I had to do the lifting and bending; my mother could only do the weightless work. Barbara had meanwhile arrived and dispatched all the children to the outdoors. She helped me put him in the car while my mother carried down a little bag. We deposited him at the hospital and regarded each other as though we had taken part in a special test by fire.

Sensitive to my father's plea not to be submitted to further surgery or hospitalization, I was reluctant to have him admitted again. Marcure had persuaded me, however, that what was involved was only the relief of pain and that it was essential in order to honor my father's mandate, accepted by the family, to move towards death in as easy a manner as remained possible. He assured me that it could not be done at home.

Subsequently my father was given an intrathecal infusion of absolute alcohol—an injection of sensation-dulling alcohol into the sacral nerves at the base of the spine. It did serve to relieve the bladder spasms then causing him the worst pain and therefore was, I believe, the right thing to do. The loss of bowel and bladder control normally expected from this procedure had already occurred.

For the week he was in the hospital, we did our best to give my mother some distraction and fun. She had barely left my father's side, not to speak of the house, in the three months since the trip to Florida. At first she would go only to private places like our Stockbridge Bowl cottage. Then we convinced her to accompany us to Tanglewood, where she had resisted going out of a double disinclination to visit a familiar haunt without her husband and to cope with the many friends she could expect to meet there. We took a picnic supper before the concert and sat on the lawn looking down to Stockbridge Bowl, a typically lovely Berkshire summer tableau. Friends did approach but graciously so, imposing no strain of explanation or reportage on my mother.

Through the week, she paid regular calls on my father at the hospital, hearing out both his complaints about the noises in the corridor and his paeans of praise for the nurses constantly gliding into his room. But she sat long at dinner with us, too, sampling widowhood, so to speak. Of her own illness she rarely spoke. "Oh, I have a touch of cancer," she had once lightly told Jayn. She had stopped receiving the particular chemotherapy to which she'd had such a fierce reaction. She looked a bit thin but otherwise well, and she took extra sun.

My father came home from the hospital for the last week in August—our last week at Stockbridge. He could not manage stairs. He was now bedridden. The folds on his face largely defeated my efforts to shave him with his electric razor. His catheter, hooked to a bag hanging at bedside, could not be concealed as it snaked out from under the bedclothes, and it added to our hesitation to let the children into the room for daily greetings. But we decided that in this as in other medical matters, calm explanations could soften harsh facts. The children expressed only mild curiosity and no embarrassment at the scene. They spoke in normal tones around my parents and saved their squeals and tussles for other times.

In only a few days, however, the heavy pain seeped back. The mass of the cancer was expanding beyond the area served by the deadened nerve roots. How grossly unfair that the cancer should be skipping ever out of the moving reach of medicine, I thought. Was intense pain for a shorter period the price an old person had to pay for avoiding a gentler debility/senility over a longer time?

Dr. Mamonas, back in town, came over on the day before we were to return to Washington. He poked my father briefly and indicated he could do nothing more than prescribe drugs for pain.

I walked out with him to his car. "Don't you doctors have something you can just give people in this condition?" I asked. My father had suffered enough, I went on; he was not quitting early; he had earned rest.

Tersely Dr. Mamonas replied that he was doing everything he could to make my father's remaining time bearable. And since no "heroic measures" were being administered, none could be withdrawn.

Later I realized that I could not have known whether he had taken my urging to foreshorten the end. No layman could know and, in those circumstances—a lone doctor attending an obviously terminal patient—no professional would be likely to know. It came to my attention that in one survey of 660 internists, more than forty per cent said they would increase dosages of narcotics, knowing that it would not only ease pain but bring on fatal respiratory arrest.

But in my father's instance, I do not believe this could have happened. For when I called on Dr. Mamonas after my father died, he reported that he had just been reading Socrates on death—specifically, on the theme that life is a prison. Too good to be true, I thought: a Greek doctor reading Greek philosophy. We talked about it a bit. He struck me as too solid, too literal to help a dying person "break out." I was confused when I left his office, but I was to learn much more of the intricate layers of values involved in such terminal situations when my mother's time came. My father's case turned out to be, by comparison, relatively clear-cut.

Taking my turn in the Rosenfeld children's rotation, I came back up to Pittsfield alone for a weekend late in September. Drugs and deterioration had almost completely suppressed any inclination on my father's part to complain of his condition, or to participate in life at all. A year previous, he had underlined in *The Lives of a Cell* a quotation of Thomas Browne's: "The long habit of living indisposeth us to dying." Now the habit had been broken. He slept most of the day; the difference between night and day had been obliterated. He rarely spoke. His arms and legs were thin as a Bengali beggar's. He sipped Coke through a straw to make the paste needed to get down the pills. My mother emptied the catheter bag two or three times a day, flushing away his sickness and his lifeblood.

There was scarcely any possibility left of communication with him. I thought that at least I might say as a final word that I loved him, something I had never said directly to either parent, something I felt would complete my filial obligation to him and indicate as well that I had passed into a new realm of personal liberation. But, feeling a tightness, I held back, the drag of two lifetimes' (his and mine) custom of restraint denying the beckoning rewards of release.

My father was beyond such self-indulgent tugs of war. At my coming and going he merely murmured, "Stevie."

I was leaving for Washington. My mother, hovering at bedside, was staying to the end. Die quickly, I said in silence to the crumpled face on the pillow.

EIGHT

Funeral

MY FATHER had wanted to die at home, where only about one in five Americans now dies, and he did, in the hours before dawn on Tuesday, October 21, 1975, a bright, cool Berkshire-autumn day. My mother was sleeping in one of the side-by-side twin beds with which they had replaced their old double bed at the onset of his decline. Behind them was the double headboard filled with his bird's nest of books, notebooks, eyeglass cases, music programs, and children's drawings: clues to the contemporary life. Atop the bureau, leaning on the facing wall, were the formal photos of his parents and her parents: evidence of roots.

She awoke during the night and lay tense for hours, straining to detect sound or movement from the figure a few inches away, unable to bring herself to put on a light and confirm what her alarm told her had taken place. Only after dawn did she call doctor and undertaker and then, the body removed, phone her children, first Jayn.

I was at breakfast. Her voice wavered but held. "Oh, Mom," I said. "I'm sorry." I cried. Barbara came to me, as did the children, uncertain in the ways of grief. The picture of my mother alone in an empty house bore in and I telephoned one of her closest Pittsfield friends, herself a widow, to ask her to go over, which she did at once.

Anticipating the 400-mile funeral trek, we had replaced our failing station wagon two weeks earlier. I had shined up my good shoes. For the hour or two before we could leave, we sent the children off to their schools. David, we later found out, could not bring himself to explain the particular reason why he would be absent for the rest of the week, even though he needed that sort of good excuse in order still to get a part in a class play. I conducted a round-robin exchange on the phone with my siblings, and called a few friends. The death on schedule of a sick limp man of eighty, one who has lived a rich life and is at peace, is no tragedy but the event itself was dully jarring. The touching with family and friends drew the sting away.

One friend's response was strangely cool. Later he wrote: "For ten days I had been in bed with pneumonia and the morning of your call was the first time I had been well enough to come downstairs for breakfast. I was unable to react. Forgive me." I did.

When we arrived in Pittsfield at the end of that day, the family was gathering, friends of my parents were dropping off casseroles and cakes, the house swarmed. My mother looked pale but composed, an island of detachment. I said something to her. She squeezed me back. Her eyes were piercing, blue. I had the feeling that no strength could now be drawn from our relationship that had not long ago been built into it.

We swept into the dining room for one of Alma's feasts. I took my father's place at the head of the table. Peter sat protectively close to my mother at the foot. The children were strung like pearls in between. The conversation expanded. A verbal map was drawn of the interstate highways and Berkshire cutoffs by which we'd all come "home." The children tried to spy the routes on the big framed world map on the wall—my father had hunted down a map that broke in mid-Atlantic to follow more easily the Pacific part of World War II. Somebody recalled that "Daddy" always liked the lemon pie dessert. More wine was poured. My mother smiled. I wondered if any accumulation of life and lore in my own generation could ever create that same sense of place and family centrality in the house in a post-war

Washington suburb in which I had lived only ten years.

From Washington that morning I had called the Meehan Funeral Home and dutifully issued the instructions my father had presented me in Florida. In Pittsfield I discovered that the order for cremation had been countermanded by my mother. I hesitated to raise the matter. My suspicion was that either she could not countenance the actual destruction of her husband's body or she had been persuaded to forego cremation on religious grounds. For traditionally Jews compare a corpse to an impaired Torah scroll which, though no longer usable, retains its holiness, and regard cremation as a desecration.

The facts, however, turned out to be very different. My father had evidently agreed to cremation only with great reluctance, because my mother had insisted on it for herself (for reasons unknown) and he could not bear the thought of lying alone in the cemetery without her. But the morning he died, she decided that since his real wish was to be buried, she would be buried, too. There was time to have Peter call the funeral home to make the change. It was a minuet of mutual sensibility expressing the essence of their marital style.

The two younger children we left on South Mountain Road early the next afternoon when we set out for the funeral. David and Becky, eleven and ten, we brought with us in respect to the impulse that had led Solon to comment to the effect that every Greek knew who his

grandfather was and wanted to be buried by his grandchildren. Hundreds of people were streaming into Temple Anshe Amunim's box of brick. "A lot of people
coming for Daddy," we said to my mother. The extended family, including in-laws and cousins, crowded
into Rabbi Harold Salzmann's study for the traditional
blessing of mourner's ribbons for the widow and children. The rabbi chanted gravely, his mood noticeably
heavier than our own.

He produced an embossed mouse-nibbled scrapbook
which, he reported, had been given to him some years
earlier by my father's sister Ruby. Two of her three
children were in the room and they said in surprise
they'd never seen it. Inside the front cover was the
scrawled signature of Zeno Rosenfeld, the brother of
Ruby and Jay who'd run away from home in his teens.
The first page bore a picture of a "New Senator from
Oregon," Joseph Simon, whose election (in 1898) was
noted in an adjacent clipping, "Hebrews in Public
Life."

Flicking the pages, which evidently had been pasted
up subsequently by Ruby, we saw clippings and me-
mentoes of Rosenfeld family events. There was a newspaper story we'd heard only brief reference to before:
"RESCUED FROM WATERY GRAVE: Albert Mac-
Arthur Dives Seven Times to the Bottom of the Stein-
kill Dam and Brings Little Jay Rosenfeld to the Surface—Doctors Work Hours for His Life." All of us

oohed and aahed, warmed and brought together by this chance descent into the family past.

There were some twenty of us—a pleasing bulk, I felt—in the family group that entered the sanctuary at two. The crowd had overflowed into a rear area usually opened only for holiday services. Light from a big skylight flooded the space, making it almost gay. My mother sat between Jayn and me, on the center aisle only a few feet from the flag-draped casket. Though my father had resigned from the American Legion in 1959 to protest the color bar in its Forty and Eight society, a Legion flag had nonetheless found its way to his casket. We directed my mother's attention to the single flower display she had decided to permit despite my father's no-flowers edict: a lovely design shaped like a G clef and mounted on a music stand, done by a friend with her own greenhouse.

Jayn and I glanced back and told my mother some of the people who were there. "There's John Persip," I said—a gentle black man, a caterer, wearing his Legion cap, in whose tacit name my father had resigned from the Legion.

She nodded.

"There's Pete Aulisi"—a retired tailor who had worked in my father's store for forty years. A few months later, Peter Aulisi, eighty-three, featured in an *Eagle* story as perhaps "the oldest altar boy in the world," said: "Jay was the heart of the store. I could cry when I think of him. I would like to put a little earth on his coffin and say, 'O, terra, non pesare su di lei / Perche non pesava su di te.' You understand, no? It means, 'O earth, don't be too heavy on him, he was never too heavy on you.' "

We reported another arrival. "Don't let him near me!," my mother whispered back hoarsely. "Every time he sees me on the street, he wants to kiss me, a big wet kiss, and I have to cross to the other side."

Jayn and I fought to keep from laughing aloud. "OK, Mom!"

From behind the front curtain came a cello's tones. It was, of course, Peter, a professional musician who had taken up the career my father had put down. He had chosen the Sarabande from Bach's Suite no. 2 for unaccompanied cello. My father had often played unaccompanied Bach himself, and this piece was slow and in a minor key (D). Peter's performance was intense and sculptured, an expression of my father's own musical values. I thought to myself, Peter has never played better.

The rabbi led prayers. Recalling that my father, for all his professed devoutness, could not read Hebrew, I felt passing regret that I, though not devout, had not retained my bar-mitzvah boy's Hebrew. The moment for the eulogy came. I did not know just what quotations my father had prepared to be read in place of it. Wistfully, almost as though he suspected my father had contrived to rob him of a significant occasion, the rabbi explained my father's mandate and began to read:

"The trees which I have planted here are thriving; they were once so small that I provided them with shade when I stood between them and the sun. Now, giving this shade back to me, they protect my old age as I have protected their youth."

This was from Chateaubriand's memoirs. A murmur ran through the temple.

> "Steadily, tranquilly, cheerfully,
> He finished the voyage of life.
> 'I trim myself to the storm of time,
> I man the rudder, reef the sail,
> Obey the voice at eve obeyed at prime:
> 'Lowly faithful, banish fear,
> Right onward drive unharmed;
> The port, well worth the cruise, is near,
> And every wave is charmed.' "

These lines, I later found, were from a stanza of Emerson's "Terminus" whose third line, omitted by my father, reads, "As the bird trims her to the gale, . . ."

"I make no excuses for the trouble I give you because I feel you take pleasure in obliging me."

From the British actress Sarah Siddons, who died in 1831. At this quotation, people in the pews laughed softly.

"I can die smiling."

Guillaume Apollinaire's epitaph.

The rabbi read Byron's "Were My Bosom As False As Thou Deem'st It To Be," from his *Hebrew Melodies*, concluding:

> "I have lost for that faith more than thou canst bestow,
> As the God who permits thee to prosper doth know;
> In his hand is my heart and my hope—and in thine
> The land and the life which for him I resign."

The next three selections were dedicated in my father's notes "To Beth":

> "And when—if ever—I awake
>   In a celestial sphere,
> I ask no greater happiness
>   Than that she gives me here."

This was from Hudson Maxim, the American inventor.

> ". . . in my heart
> There is a vigil, and these eyes but close
> To look within . . ."

From Byron's *Manfred*.

> "So let us melt, and make no noise,
>   No teare-floods, nor sigh-tempests move,
> T'were prophanation of our joyes
>   To tell the layetie our love."

From Donne's "A Valediction Forbidding Mourning." The congregation was somber now, entranced.

"I am sure it must be consolatory to you, and all who love me, to see how comfortably I am coming to my end."

This line, from British writer Daniel George's "Pleasant Deaths" (a chapter in his *A Book of Anecdotes*), perceptibly lightened the mood.

"What you have inherited from your mother and father, you must earn in order to possess."

From Goethe's *Faust*—the translation was my father's.

Time hung still. The people listening were half suspended by the sentiment, half tipping into delight at my father's orchestration of the scene. I was touched by yet a third consideration—that in death, through words of his own choice if not composition, he had found a way to make an authentic statement about himself, to deliver a will distributing his emotional and spiritual assets, so to speak.

These personal feelings were, in fact, on a very different wavelength from the service ethic—the Schweitzer ethic—which had guided him in his public role. I call it the Schweitzer ethic because its purest expression came in a quotation from Albert Schweitzer of which I subsequently found half a dozen copies on cards in his files.

"It is an uncomfortable doctrine which the true ethic whispers in my ear," Schweitzer wrote. "You are happy, it says; therefore you are called upon to give much. Whatever more than others you have received in health, natural gifts, working capacity, success, a beautiful childhood, harmonious family circumstances, you must not accept as being a matter of course. You must pay a price for them. You must show more than an ordinary devotion to life." This was in effect the public Jay Rosenfeld whom the hundreds in the Temple had come to honor: the man of "instinctive courtesy" and civic rectitude—a man not, I suppose, without a touch of sanctimony.

But the private man—the person alone facing death, the vulnerable husband and father—had instead been revealed. He had preempted a rabbi's eulogy, foregone a sermon of his own (for that is what the Schweitzer citation or some variant would have been), and offered as clear a distillation as was within his reach of what was personally most important to him. That, I thought, is what a father finally owes a son. I forgave him everything.

My mother, beautifully brave, led us out. None of us wanted to ride in the black limousines so she got in Jayn's and Jerry's little Peugeot to drive to the cemetery. Barbara and I picked up Dick and Kitty Cunningham, who'd come up from New York. Dick, a painter, had grown up on South Mountain Road and had gone to Harvard with my brother Rick and me. He was chortling with fine relish at the funeral's fidelity to the best spirit of our family. As my father died, I had found it difficult, as perhaps many people do, to share the experience with a lot of the people I knew. With friends like the Cunninghams, however, hesitation

yielded easily to feeling and banter. They were precisely the people I wanted in the car.

I had seen a retired Rosenfeld's employee at the funeral, Harold Depew, and it reminded me of one of my
father's favorite stories. Harold would say to a customer
entering when he, Harold, was busy, "My assistant,
Bill Blackburn, will be glad to take care of you," and a
furious Bill, Harold's senior in service, would silently
mouth the words "You son of a bitch!" Our car, lights
on, went up North Street through the red lights in the
time-honored manner of Pittsfield funeral processions.
We were roaring.

We buried my father in the Rosenfeld family plot
acquired when the Temple had first bought its own big
lot, "two rods wide and twenty rods deep," in the Pittsfield Cemetery in 1871. Integrated in life, the people of
Pittsfield, a typical New England city, had long since
segregated themselves ethnically in death.

We four Rosenfeld children clustered around our
mother. She looked infinitely tired. She had said not a
word to us about her sensation of loss, had barely cried.
Just as she had always muffled her sneezes, so she con-
tained what had to be the emotional tumult within her.
I found myself wanting her to let go.

But I had nothing left to let go myself. I had antici-
pated and accepted my father's death months earlier,
written him off. To see his casket lowered into a hard-
edged hole only made me impatient to flee the ceme-

tery, a chilly place in the flat October light. David and Becky, somewhat intimidated by their first brush with adults mumbling in mourning, huddled near us, David suspending his customary quest for cool, Becky very subdued.

"Let's go, big guys," I said. We drove back down North Street, this time—since we were not in a procession—stopping for the lights. My eyes sought out my father's old store, since renamed.

At home, close friends trooped in for memorial prayers. Three pals of my mother had organized a spread, in the Jewish community tradition. Jimmy and Mike went up to my mother, who was sitting uneasily in her chair, and draped themselves softly on her arms, one on either side. My mother was a twin, I am a twin, I have twins; in addition, as I had learned—oddly enough—only towards my father's end, his mother had a twin who died at birth. I have not been one for making much of the accident of twinhood but on that occasion I looked at our boys framing my mother and thought that that was exactly what twins were for.

She was drained and could not stay downstairs for the day's last prayers, which—after everything—were providing diminishing returns for all of us. We propelled her upstairs. Peter had hustled my father's bed out of their bedroom the previous day, and Jayn had bought a bright new skirt to clothe the mattress on my mother's. Her doctor knocked her out.

Barbara and I hung around for a few more days. I walked on South Mountain with my mother, noticing how fatigue had cramped the head-down, arm-swinging gait that had made her instantly recognizable to drivers approaching several hundred yards away. She wanted someone to help her get started on the legal and logistical matters that had to be tended to. She had me clean out my father's clothes and get rid of his vials of pills. We arranged for a nice level-headed high school senior who lived next door to sleep overnight at 173, after the family was gone, to put my mother at greater ease in a house in which she'd never lived alone.

I did enough of these chores to feel only a slight twinge of guilt when, at week's end, we left my mother and drove swiftly back to Washington—in order to go to a fancy party. I wore my mourner's ribbon and wondered why I was there.

NINE

Cancer

THIRTY YEARS AGO, for the symptoms that first alerted my mother to her impending sickness, "exploratory surgery" might have been performed and her cancer detected and removed, Dr. Joseph Budnitz, an honest and humble man, suggested after she died. As it was, diagnosis had to await a succession of exhaustive and exhausting tests which did not find suspicious traces of cancer until it had already spread "extensively" from its source in the colon to the liver and nearby lymph nodes.

Though reluctant to second-guess professionals, especially professionals who were devoted family friends, I wondered resentfully for some months if other or more frequent testing would have made a difference. Eventually I came to accept that the patient's endurance and the hospital's and doctors' resources, as well as the nature of the tests themselves, imposed certain restrictions which could not lightly be brushed away. In September 1974, for instance, a highly touted New York specialist had found and removed a polyp from the colon, without diagnosing cancer. But whether such small growths are signals of a potential malignancy is a matter of lingering medical controversy, my mother's Pittsfield cancer specialist, Dr. Jesse Spector, reported. There is no known specific test for cancer. Nearly a dozen doctors looked her over. We of the family ended up feeling certain that she had the best available care.

Meanwhile her symptoms—nausea, rectal bleeding, anemia—persisted. On February 25, 1975, the LDH count—lactic dehydrogenase is a liver enzyme—showed up as 374, against a norm below 200. "That gives you the willies," said Dr. Ralph Zupanec, her surgeon. A barium enema (her second) on March 3 picked up a lesion, or structural injury, in the mid-transverse colon. Surgery on March 10 located a cancer so extensive that only a "somewhat limited" removal of tissue could be done. "At this point she was in trouble," Dr. Zupanec later said. A "general practitioner of surgery," he had settled in a small city in order to be involved in the life of his patients. "There is no known way to eradicate the disease. It could go from weeks to years—there are all different sorts."

Liver cancer is a "bad cancer," Dr. Spector told me. "It grows quietly before the symptoms appear and so by the time it's discovered it's big and evasive." Moreover, if it's secondary or metastatic, meaning it has spread from somewhere else in the body, then things are worse, for one is dealing with a cancer that is in the bloodstream and may spread still further.

Only in the last few years has evidence been developed that chemotherapy, beyond sometimes making cancer patients feel better, in some cases helps them live longer, though it does not cure the disease. For my mother's kind of cancer, treatment by certain drugs used in combination—drugs previously used separately—has allowed perhaps one out of two patients to live, say, seven or eight months longer than they otherwise would. She was given methyl, a compound with cancer-suppressing potential, and 5-fluorouracil, an antimetabolite.

Through the spring and summer, she did well. The wound of her surgery had healed enough by May to permit the trip to Florida, and by August she was not only tending to my father under heavy circumstances but playing a little tennis. To the methyl, however, she had such a brutal reaction—nausea and vomiting so wracking that I was genuinely glad never to be an actual witness—that treatments with this chemical had to be spaced out. When I told Jesse Spector how traumatized the family had been by her reaction to the methyl, he said that it was a reasonable price to pay for a lengthened life. But he conceded that he had not apprehended how difficult it is to see a loved one in agony until he had seen his own wife in the clutches of a toothache not too long before.

A liver scan in September showed that my mother's cancer was "progressive" and she was taken off 5-fluorouracil and put on mitomycin C, a tissue destroyer. She continued, nonetheless, to feel all right, which Spector attributed to three considerations. She was preoccupied with her husband. She was not as sick as others with the same disease. And "She came across as a lovely person. She was a strong person. She had it together."

This was the state of affairs when my father died in October. We eyed my mother anxiously, aware that her emotions, like her cancer, played out of view. A day or two after the funeral, Dr. Budnitz took me aside. He said he wanted us children to know that my mother, deprived now by her husband's death of the principal source of her own will to live, could well herself go into a decline. We should not be surprised.

As I was later to learn, Dr. Spector had scant sympathy for the theory that such a thing as the will to live could affect the progress of a cancer. By biofeedback, a person could will changes in heartbeat or could control certain other muscles as in belly dancing or transcendental meditation, he conceded, "but this won't alter the kinetics of cell growth." Said Spector, then thirty-three: "I'm a research doctor. Show me."

"I can't," said Budnitz, a cardiologist and GP of almost twice that age when, on another occasion, I relayed this viewpoint back to him, "but that's to emphasize just things that are measureable. Some things aren't."

On that post-funeral October day, however, he simply warned in his soft, wincing way that my mother was entering a dangerous period. He had known my parents closely for more than a quarter century. It pained him to bear a dark forecast. I took him very seriously and quietly spread the word.

My mother had never inquired about her prognosis from any of her doctors. She never even asked what had caused her cancer. She never lamented or cursed it. Throughout her illness she chose to live in the present and to maintain her normal positive and outgoing attitude. Neither Budnitz nor we children thought it made sense to inform her of his forecast.

Her twin sister Frances, from New York, decided to stay in Pittsfield for a week after we children left. That was a tonic: with Francie she set about replying to the hundreds of condolence notes. I eventually went through them all myself and was touched especially by intimate notes from new younger people in the county whom I was not even aware my parents knew. Every day she walked with Francie. For Barbara's and my anniversary, just one week after my father's death, she remembered to write, enclosing a keepsake postcard from Dettelbach, the town where my grandfather had been born.

My mother reviewed and confirmed her earlier decision to stay in Pittsfield, knowing that Jayn and I were both prepared to take her in. Things never got to the point where Barbara and I actually sat down to plan for the event, though I had begun to mentally rearrange the living space in our house. For my mother's sake as well as ours, I am glad she never came.

First consulting us, my mother invited Syd Pincu, the widow who had gone to her the morning my father died, to move into the big South Mountain Road house. Syd gently said no, realizing that the keeping of a certain distance would serve their friendship better. My mother also thought through, and rejected, the idea of moving her bedroom downstairs into the snug little "new room." She wanted continuity. These were necessary and useful exercises to test her command of her new circumstances. Too, they gave us children a taste of our own enhanced advisory role.

Back in Washington, I felt—for a while, acutely—wistful and chastened, somehow a better person, now a member of a community to which I had not belonged before. I wrote the people in Pittsfield who had shown special kindness to our family, and read the letters that had come to me. Some of these letters recalled the writer's own association with my father. Others portrayed him as someone who had expanded the writers' notion of what many kinds of fathers were possible. Still other letters, written by people who knew me but not him, reflected on the writers' inheritance from their own fathers. There was no pattern, but among these letters and among the words spoken to me personally by friends and acquaintances, there was a respect for the event of losing one's father and a pervading sense that it was a compass-setting time.

Many of those who addressed me proceeded, without pausing, to relate episodes from the death of their own parents. A swift intimacy could be established in these exchanges, even in one instance with a foreign ambassador whose government I had just harshly attacked in a *Post* editorial. In virtually the same mail he wrote me a graceful personal note and sent the newspaper an outraged public reply to the editorial. I resolved to try to be more attentive, beyond the bounds of normal courtesy, to the still-living parents of my contemporaries.

When, soon, my black lapel ribbon somehow disappeared, I shrugged.

Chick Budnitz phoned one night in mid-November to state that my mother was getting around well enough but was in something of a depression. She had spent the better part of two years pinned in the house, the last months pinned in one room with her dying husband, and she needed a change of scene. We had hoped to launch her on a routine of family rounds and so it was arranged among the children that she would visit the New York outposts starting on Thanksgiving. Elated, we figured to get her down to Washington, and then perhaps to Florida a month later.

With all that in prospect, she appeared much cheered when I went up alone to Pittsfield on November 15. I took her out to dinner at the home of Helen and Bob Maislen and we had lunch with the Lipskys the next day. She wrote me after I left, enclosing a check for the air fare ("I know you can afford it but I want to do it," she always insisted) and declaring, "You just can't know how healing it was to have you here this weekend."

Ann Salzarulo, the girl next door who was holding down the fort at night, was awakened by a knock at 4:30 A.M. on November 21. My mother was breathing hard and rubbing her chest with shaking hands. Ann phoned Dr. Spector, who ordered her taken to the emergency room. "Oh, dear, oh, dear," said my mother as Ann put on shoes and coat against the night's snow and inched her down to the garage. At the hospital, Ann waited until the nurses called her in about eight. "Please phone Jayn," said my mother, crushing Ann with a smile.

She was admitted for an acute myocardial infarction,

or heart attack, evidently brought on by cumulative stress and perhaps also by cancer-induced anemia—the blood being conducted to the heart carried inadequate oxygen.

"It was unfair," Herb Glodt later said to me. "Just as she was on her way back up," rued Chick Budnitz, who did not have to remind me of his dark forecast of the previous month.

It was during these days, which happened to coincide with a harrowing *Post* labor-management dispute in which I'd been peripherally involved, that Barbara and I were jolted awake by a phone call at 4:30 A.M. "Stephen Rosenfeld?" a harsh voice said—it was no doctor. "We're going to break your legs and burn your house down." One of the striking unions had spoken. I felt almost relieved.

And in the hospital the situation got worse. Agents in the tissue-destroying drug she was taking for her cancer apparently had damaged the lining of some blood vessels and she developed an infected ulceration of a vein, or phlebitis, at the point where a needle transfusing blood and glucose-salt had entered the back of her left hand. It gave her intense pain for days to a degree that no other aspect of her sickness, the bursts of extreme nausea excepted, ever did. I ached at seeing her so distracted and my mind flashed back to stories about how Richard Nixon's phlebitis had itself brought him near death.

I returned to Pittsfield on December 6 to take her home, carrying her up the stairs with a disconcerting ease. She volunteered tersely that she would refuse to return to the hospital. The removal from home over-whelmed in her mind the convenience of care. The wound on her hand seemed open to the bone.

On December 10 she suffered a relapse—in effect, said Budnitz, the completion of her first heart attack. He treated her at home and she soon picked up. On December 26, however, for chest pains (angina) and general weakness, Glodt, in Budnitz's absence, put her back in the hospital, in the coronary care unit. Budnitz took over again on December 29, and removed her from the unit. He changed the treatment of her phlebitis from wet to dry, ending the soaking.

"Why am I so weak?," she asked him.

He figured it was mostly anemia induced by her cancer, and gave her two blood transfusions. She felt a bit stronger. Her hand began to heal.

Barbara and I and the children, for their December recess, arrived the day after she entered the hospital. Ever upbeat, my mother had bought herself a season's pass at Bousquet's, the ski area a mile up the road. We converted it into a week's ski school tickets for the kids.

The shuttlecock treatment my mother was receiving between the two doctors somewhat confused us, though we knew it stemmed from necessities of their own schedules and vacations. They in turn were sensitive to

our confusion and, as professionals and as fast friends of
my mother, were prepared to leave her in the care of
one of them—Budnitz, the cardiologist—as logistics
permitted.

But this was of passing moment. What gnawed at us
deeply was the knowledge that on account of her heart
trouble my mother's chemotherapy had had to be suspended. This meant that her cancer, only partially re-
strained before, was now running free. The anemia,
which was making her feel sick and weak and drowsy,
was the red flag. Even as Budnitz explained to me the
need for chemotherapy, however, he acknowledged its
cost. "It's poison," he said tersely with a snap of his
head—capable of destroying good tissue as well as bad.
My head spun.

A pine cone decorated by Becky hung over my
mother's hospital bed. She asked about the children's
ski lessons. Were we being taken care of well by Alma?
She lavished praise on the nurses for their personal
kindness, which had dispelled her reluctance to return
to the hospital. How much old people in hospitals fear
the manipulation of strangers, I reflected.

On January 2, 1976, a Friday, we brought her home.
She brightened. Jayn had arrived with her family.
Together we interviewed a dozen or more women to
find the right nurse's aide or licensed practical nurse.
My mother now needed the extra home care. Rose Bud-
nitz, Chick's wife, called excitedly to report that the

death that day of a neighbor had freed up a particularly good nurse's aide. "It's not even in the paper yet!" she exulted.

Sherry Nolan, a pretty, well-rounded, dark-haired woman in her twenties, seemed to have just the right experience and uncluttered personality. We hired her on the spot.

"No," I said, when not a week later Sherry phoned to relay that my mother had contracted pneumonia. It had resulted from her cancer or chemotherapy—both the disease and the treatment can reduce one's capacity to combat infections—or perhaps it was just going around. Budnitz put the heaviest onus on the chemotherapy for knocking out the white corpuscles which attack germs. The pneumonia savaged her. And it further extended the time when the chemotherapy could be resumed.

"This is unfair," she told a friend, in a brief rare complaint.

Another blood transfusion was ordered. Sherry passed that word in a late-evening call which I took in our bedroom. Barbara was in the shower and I said, over the sound of the water, "I think she'll die by April."

"Oh, honey. Why?"

"The winter is too long."

For my father had groaned about the length of the preceding winter and had died in October before facing another, and my mother had gritted her teeth heading into this one alone.

That weekend I went up to see her. It was dismal. Budnitz, on his daily call, wrote in his notes: "Terrible day today. Slept most of time. Steve is home and she hardly knows him. Has no orientation re time of day. This morning she is asleep, but trembling and a chill." And the next day: "Liver is enlarged . . . tender."

I was leaving Monday on the 7:30 A.M. flight from the nearby Pittsfield airport to LaGuardia. The previous evening I had told Sherry, who ordinarily would have stayed the night, to go off and to come back at seven. I awoke and dressed, hearing nothing, and went into my mother's room a few minutes before seven to say good-bye. Her bed was empty. I rushed into her bathroom. She was lying twisted on her back on the narrow space of tile between the toilet and the wall, her nightgown hiked high around her waist.

I thought: she is dead because I let Sherry go. But she was alive. I put her in bed. Sherry came up the stairs at that minute, saying that my airport cab was waiting. I felt hopelessly guilty for running off but, with Sherry there, could see no good reason to stay.

Later in the day, in New York, I arranged with his secretary to speak with Budnitz on the phone that evening at seven. No sooner had the arrangement been made than I was granted my requested appointment with the Secretary General of the United Nations at . . . seven. Journalistic duty called. But I could not, even in the symbolic form of a phone appointment with her doctor, set my mother aside once more on that exploding day. I sent Kurt Waldheim my apologies and, from the U.N., called Chick Budnitz. My mother had suffered a second bout of pneumonia. Only months later did I inform Budnitz of the choice I'd made. "You shouldn't have," he said quietly, smiling.

Two weeks later Budnitz told Jayn that prompt resumption of chemotherapy was the only way to halt my mother's progressive wasting. Jayn vigorously agreed, since it no longer made sense to worry that chemotherapy itself might be wasting. Thus the whole Christmas vacation issue of balancing off the pluses and minuses of the treatment was resolved by the advance of the disease. I repeated Jayn's accounting to Barbara and went to another room to be alone, feeling not so much sad as pained that my mother was dying. So two and a half months after chemotherapy had first been suspended, she returned to her cancer specialist. Dr. Spector found her "obviously jaundiced"—evidence of a failing liver—and pronounced her "beyond chemotherapy."

Except that that was not the way it was initially reported to me.

The doctors figured it would help Sherry Nolan to maintain her customary sunny disposition, which they regarded as therapeutic in itself, if they told her only the bare facts: treatments by injection were being replaced by prescription of a new drug to be taken orally. When I called the next morning, my mother was in the tub—a good sign. The impression I carried away from Sherry was that treatment by injections, a method my mother disliked—in the hospital at Christmas time she had begged to be spared further injections—was yielding to treatment by a method that gave her no distress. Moreover, Sherry reported, my mother was getting dressed, coming downstairs, reading the paper and mail, asking for friends—further good signs.

High on delight, I reached Barbara at her office to say that my mother's cancer had turned out to be still treatable after all. Later the same day I phoned Pittsfield again to speak with my mother directly. I alerted her that I'd be appearing that afternoon on a National Public Radio program she often listened to. She seemed groggy and I was unsure she'd understood the message. But that night as I walked in the door, Jimmy pointed eagerly to Barbara, who was talking on the phone. "It's Grandma," he said. She wanted to say how much she'd liked my radio appearance.

"The old Jewish mother!," I said to Barbara. We exchanged her usual scotch and my bourbon for martinis for the occasion.

In fact, as Chick Budnitz soon let us know, she had been shifted from chemotherapy to prednisone, a drug administered simply to keep up appetite and spirits and to suppress certain symptoms. The end was now in sight. My brother Peter said what we all felt—that it was good she was not in pain as my father had been. I fled from contemplation of her decay and turned on the television to watch the winter Olympics.

Prednisone

FOR THIRTEEN YEARS of marriage Barbara and I had been unable to keep straight that 401 was the area code for telephoning her parents in Cranston, Rhode Island, and 413 the code for calling mine in Pittsfield. It became a family joke. But now, by the frequency of our calls to Pittsfield, we fixed on the difference. Sherry Nolan usually answered, though we had rigged an extension to the bedroom lounge chair which was increasingly coming to mark the outer circle—only intermittently reached—of my mother's daily routine.

Most of the time, day and night, she was sleeping, or

drifting under the surface of consciousness, beyond being disturbed by the ring. If she was awake, she might briefly take the receiver. We stopped asking her how she felt and mostly just provided her with a quick rundown on family doings. "Love to the children," she would say. Then Sherry, having trotted downstairs, would come on and post medical bulletins, social notes, and other items of the day. It tickled me as a journalist to be hanging on Sherry's every word with an intensity surpassing the closest attentions I expected from my own readers. Sherry had, in fact, a good journalist's way of answering concisely, to the limits of her information, the questions I had on my mind.

It was surprising how changeable, within certain tightening limits, my mother's condition was. Some days she would barely get out of bed, others she might go downstairs for the afternoon. These daily variations produced in me, I think, a certain detachment about her fate. She was "dying," but far from that being a predictable process for which one could plan as for a journey on an interstate highway, it turned out to be a process proceeding, as it were, on an unimproved country road.

At first I tended to project each zig and zag to its extreme. It was hard, if she faltered on Monday, not to think she would weaken more on Tuesday. It was tempting, if she rallied on Wednesday, to hope that she would rally further on Thursday. I even found myself feeling uncharitably impatient on occasion to learn that her condition was rather stable. It was an unnerving absence of clues.

But my daily perceptions began to flatten out. Feeling "better" came to be increasingly relative: not much more than emerging from a few days' feverish fog into a thick-voiced moment of conversation on the phone, or managing to stay awake long enough to receive a brief visit from friends. People said, sympathetically, that they hoped things would "clear up" or "get better," by which they meant, of course, that the tension if not the distress of her situation and mine would yield to her death. But as the weeks wore on, I did not feel overwhelming tension or distress. Nor did I regard my mother's situation as being a fight against death, or even a drama. I took it as a cumulative layering of consciousness and experience, proceeding in my case by occasional spurts of concentrated sadness relieved by longer terms of preoccupation with normal affairs.

Time is cut into ever smaller segments for the dying and for those who attend them. Dying does not stop time but articulates the flow. It does not universalize experience but conveys an ever sharper sense of the particular. I learned that, especially on the long-distance phone.

By common consent my sister Jayn had become the traffic director, assuring a steady flow of Rosenfeld children's visits to Pittsfield. My mother's sister Francie and her husband, Bud Cantr, joined the pattern. Someone went up for a day or two once or twice a week so that my mother was never left long without a family caller. My father had had her in constant attendance at his deathbed. This was the least we could do for her.

In between visits, we siblings consulted with each other. Since, unlike my father, my mother was approaching death with enough mental awareness to perceive it, we asked ourselves how she felt about the end. She never explicitly provided us the materials for an answer. She asked her doctors only about specific new symptoms, such as a backache, which Budnitz felt might be evidence of cancer spreading but which he saw no purpose either in testing or trying to treat.

I had pondered for months the question of what "knowing" about death was: what was it that was actually known, on what level, with what emotional or psychological resonance? I concluded that my mother knew everything she wanted to know, in the way she wanted to know it. She was approaching death without fear or regret or pain. Our puzzlement was not reflected in any feelings we ever perceived in her. A self-supporting orphan at age fifteen, she was sustaining her independence and self-control now.

I flew up, believing it might be for the last time, the weekend of February 21–22, arriving at Hartford's Bradley Field, driving north through the tobacco fields and subdivisions in the Connecticut River valley, cutting west on the Massachusetts Turnpike to make the long climb through the hill towns, leaving the pike at

Lee and steering the familiar turns to South Mountain Road. A pleasant enough drive in any season, it afforded me the only solitude of that period—a respite I used to reflect, with a driver's flickering attention, on the scene I knew I would find at home.

My mother was sleeping on the "new room" couch, head awkwardly back, mouth slack, looking small under an afghan. I canvased the deterioration: the receding hairline, the hair itself yellowed from its previous grandmother's-white, the skin wan, the wrinkles at the eyes crumbling into desert parchment. I could circle her biceps with thumb and middle finger. She had on her red robe, a gift from Marianne and Karl Lipsky, which she wore with religious regularity as much to thank them for their kindness, I always felt, as for its warmth and color.

"Oh," she said, opening her eyes to slits. Two months earlier they had been triangles. "You're here. Have you had lunch?" I kissed her cheek. "I'm always so tired," she said, fatigue dragging her away from a moment she had had to be anticipating for hours.

Sherry was by now on duty twenty hours a day weekdays, twenty-four hours weekends. Alma Pinney relieved her and cooked dinner on weekdays. She thrived on such a heavy schedule, Sherry said convincingly. Being single and determined to make out on her own, she had recently bought her own house in Housatonic and was glad to be earning the extra money.

She had strong ideas about her work. As she told me

at lunch, she had worked in a nursing home before switching over to working in sick people's homes. "You had to take care of ten persons a shift and each week you got a new ten. If you cleared up a patient's rash, by the time you got that patient back, the rash would be back, too." In hospitals, Sherry (a nurse's aide) went on, "the registered nurses do the charts, the licensed practical nurses give medicines, and the nurse's aides do the work—the others are too 'educated' to work. My real satisfaction is taking care of one person. Some people say, 'It's terrible, you have to clean up the mess,' but I don't mind if it helps the person. Even in eight weeks," she finished up with a rush, "I've come to love your mother, Steve."

Smoking as she chatted, Sherry filled me in on the medical symptoms, the doctors' visits, the friends who'd stopped by or phoned, the menus, the pills, the draws on petty cash, the household maintenance chores needed or done—the stuff of my mother's dependency. Months earlier, thinking of the people who might be hired to tend my parents, I had imagined at best adequate, neutral servants filling in the intervals and duties left by family members and old friends. A depressing number of lonely and garrulous women had applied for the job. I had never imagined anyone either so central to my mother's existence or so perfectly suited to the role. She relieved me entirely of any incipient guilt about consigning my mother to hired care.

At night, Sherry told me, when my mother sometimes wet her bedclothes two or three times, she would change her, explaining, "Mrs. Rosenfeld, you're perspiring." She washed food-spattered robes constantly "so that she won't see that she's spilled." With a fine touch for feelings of people she barely knew, she summoned my mother's friends on her own, beading them evenly through the week. The previous weekend Francie, who had been sitting with my mother, left the room briefly, and my mother got up in a haze to go to the bathroom and fell, not hurting herself but catapulting Francie into remorse. "I told her, 'Francie, don't worry, it could happen to anyone'," Sherry related.

How unwarranted it had been, I later thought, to have kept the full facts temporarily from Sherry at the time my mother had been found to be too sick to receive further chemotherapy. The information had been withheld so that by mood if not by word my mother would not be further weighted down. But Sherry was an experienced tender to the sick who knew the sequence of dying better than any of us Rosenfeld children. And she had a fundamentally loving philosophy guiding her work which impelled her to bathe her patient in skillful consideration and not to tinge the atmosphere with negativism or, for that matter, with any cares she may have had on her own mind. Her sense of duty never lapsed.

We propped my mother up after lunch but she could not get into conversational gear.

"So tired," she whispered, fading.

Dinner was served upstairs on a tray. I sat with a drink while she laboriously chewed. Thinking that otherwise I would never know and a whole chapter in the family history would remain faint, I tried to draw her out on details of her early life that I had not known, or not known for sure, before.

Her father, who did "something in mathematics," had skipped out of Russian Lithuania to avoid army service in the Russo-Japanese war and had later sent for his wife and three daughters. I knew that. But I had not known that my mother could actually recall being in some kind of crib on the boat crossing the ocean; that it was in childbirth, or so some in the family said, that her mother had died when she was about seven; that the foster home in which she was then placed was headed by a cigar maker who spoke German in the house and whose wife rarely spoke at all—she could not recall their names.

I asked her if her own hard childhood had shaped her views about the way she wanted to conduct her own family life.

"I suppose so," she said slowly.

I paused, awaiting insight.

"I suppose so."

The weekend passed. As I left, dirty ice was melting in a February rain.

I went to a Washington Bullets basketball game the following week with, as it happened, two friends whose mother and father respectively happened also to be dying at that time. I returned warmed by our mutual awareness of each other's passage and exhilarated by the gliding play of the Bullets' Dave Bing. Sherry had called and I phoned right back. My mother was resisting getting out of bed, bathing, dressing, and so on—the rails of habit to which Sherry had had her keep hold. Her physical signs were falling.

"All she has left is her will," Barbara observed when I'd hung up.

"How long do you think it will be?" I asked. I peered into the bathroom mirror trying to pick out my mother's bone structure. There it was, I nodded contentedly, in the cheeks, around the eyes. The sudden and frightening thought occurred: I will be alone.

"What are you thinking of?" asked Barbara.

"The basketball game." It was so.

The usual hour of Sherry's next call—4 P.M.—set off its own alarm. Dr. Glodt, who had assumed my mother's care during Dr. Budnitz's absence on vacation, wanted the children informed that "the end seems imminent." She was in "something like a coma," Sherry said. Herb Glodt had ordered a halt to guests, baths and other ingredients of the engaged life, and had taken her off her antibiotics, vitamins, and sedatives. He was phasing out the prednisone.

"I'm awfully sorry, Steve," said Sherry.

"Take care of her, Sherry," I said. I was overcome.

The children soon came home from school and I snapped at David for something, even though a friend—normally a protection against parental reprisal—was there. Supper produced an impasse with Jimmy. "I'll only eat the beans if you're nice to me," he said. I felt cheap that I should be chewing up the kids. Barbara buffered as best she could.

The skies cleared the next day, a Saturday. I took the kids to "Hojo's" for ice cream and we played basketball. Barbara came home late from an all-day education meeting and we sat at the breakfast table for a supper of hot dogs and french fries. I made martinis and then poured some beer.

"We'll be going up to Pittsfield soon," I said.

"Will it be vacation time?" asked Mike.

"Of course not," said Becky, "it's not a vacation."

"It's because Grandma is very sick and dying," I said.

Becky said, "I wish she wouldn't die."

"Well, she is," injected Dave.

"Where will we go skiing, in Colorado?" (where Barbara and I had gone a month earlier) asked Mike.

"It costs too much to take you kids skiing in Colorado," I said. "Maybe we'll take you skiing at the Lipskys. Kids, I'm very sad. It makes me feel very alone to have my parents die. There's no one I can go to any more."

Barbara said, "You're lucky, you've known all four of your grandparents." She began talking of her own. The children already knew her mother's mother had lived in their house. They did not know what a crowded and difficult life it had meant for all of them. Barbara recalled her mother's father, who had a mustache and smoked foul-smelling cigars.

"Yech," said Mike. Jimmy listened attentively, in his style.

Barbara said she'd tried to teach her grandmother English in exchange for Yiddish lessons but her grandmother, who'd lived in the United States fifty years, refused to learn. She recalled that her father's father had a long beard.

Dave at once stated that my father's father had a mustache.

I asked how he knew.

"From the picture on Grandpa's bureau," he said.

Barbara, who had been named for her grandmother, said that if her family had gotten it straight in time that her grandmother's Hebrew name was not Basya (which became Barbara) but Brina, she would have been named Brina. "Who would have married me then?" she declared.

"Sounds like a pickle," I said.

"Sounds like what we're studying in school—brine shrimp," said Mike.

Everybody was laughing. I thought: this family is really clicking because Barbara picked up an idea and made it go.

"Bath time," I announced.

"Only if you play push the tush," Jimmy yelled.

On the children's corridor rug, I let each of the little boys in turn push my rear and knock me down as I stalked the other. We played bucking bronco and then a game in which I grabbed their legs and they squirmed out of my grasp and out of their pants. I shoved them into the bathtub and soaped them down, Jimmy ribless with baby fat, Mike tough like a boxer. They climbed out and clung to me. I brushed Michael's hair accidentally too hard.

"I'm dying, help, I'm dying," he shouted. "I'm dying!"

Sunday March 7 Dr. Budnitz took my mother back in tow and, to our astonishment, restored medication and activities. Jayn, arriving in expectation that she would be fading out, told me in her nice flutist's diction that she was fading back in. So elated was Jayn, in fact, that she broke off our conversation about our mother and had me hold the receiver up to a taped CBS television program, unavailable on a Pittsfield channel, on which she was playing a piccolo solo at that precise minute.

"Doesn't that stun you?" I said of the change in the treatment.

"Budnitz doesn't want to start the countdown," Jayn said.

My subsequent inquiry brought out that the two doctors had profoundly differing notions of a doctor's purpose in the final days. As Herb Glodt explained to me, "She was in a liver coma—ninety per cent of the liver cells were dead. Her personality was changing. It was time to withdraw the prednisone. It stimulates the bone marrow and gives a sense of euphoria, but it wasn't working." He went on: "Dying is no big deal. Living means *living*. An oncologist hopes for remission. He's playing the odds. But I have to take care of the whole patient. I differentiate between life and living. Living means reacting to friends and the environment, having hope. I feel strongly about this."

Chick Budnitz, on the other hand, who had seen her constantly through the winter, had returned from his vacation to find her condition "essentially unchanged." As long as she could still participate in the flow at that level, he believed, he did not want to take upon himself the decision that she should not do so. "I was doing my best under circumstances that were futile and hopeless," he said. "The comfort of a human being was my greatest concern during her last days."

Unprepared for a terminal situation which presented such apparently differing alternatives to equally conscientious practitioners, I had neither basis nor reason to judge which alternative was "better." Both were rooted in a humane respect for life and death and in love for the patient. But although the difference in terms of doctor's philosophy was considerable, the difference in terms of the actual length or quality of the patient's life was small. It was, I finally decided, not so much a medical choice, certainly not an ethical one, as one of aesthetics, a preference for one "death style" over another. I did not wish to question either decision. But I was glad that they were made in the order in which they were, mostly because of what happened in the brief period following Budnitz's return.

Jayn left Sunday. Peter drove up that evening. Rick flew in for my mother's seventieth birthday on March 8. She bathed, dressed, came downstairs, and sat at the table with friends for a birthday cake baked by Alma Pinney's daughter, quietly taking in the scene. It was a soft and rippling occasion.

I arrived not long after Rick had gone back. I handed her Becky's present, a string-on-wood design she had made herself.

"Can I eat it?" she slurred. "Do you mind if I sleep?"

ELEVEN

Home

NOT A WEEK had passed but, Chick Budnitz reported to me in Washington, my mother's capacity to take and hold food had so shriveled that to gain energy she would have to be fed intravenously. This would require entering a hospital. Budnitz did not recommend this course, he only presented it as an option. We Rosenfeld children had long ago talked out the question of extreme or artificial measures that might seem to stretch, beyond our shared sense of appropriateness, our parents' natural hold on life. In the spirit of the family consensus I reacted immediately. "No needles, no hospitals. We want her to slip out at home." I called to confirm with my brother Rick, reaching his wife Gillian, who reported their dismay that a Pittsfield friend of my mother's, also a cancer patient, had just died "all tubed up." We would not permit that for her.

I had felt for some time I wanted to be on the scene for my mother's last days. Having just participated in a decision that would probably shorten her biological life, I felt an additional measure of obligation to be with her when she died. I flew home.

Marianne Lipsky met me at the Pittsfield airport at six, and a half hour later, Karl, who'd been skiing in Vermont for the day, was dropped off at the house. The deftness of the rendezvous tickled us all. Swedish-born Marianne had brought a fresh jar of her own herring in dill sauce.

To me, my mother, eyes black and skin yellow, was dying. She stared at me intelligently but without a flicker of recognition.

Marianne, seeing with her designer's eye my mother's taut skin and shock of white hair and purity of facial bone line, said, "Beth, you are beautiful."

"Thank you," my mother said.

"Have your Coke, Mrs. Rosenfeld," Sherry Nolan said, joshing her nicely, wielding a napkin without engaging my mother's attention to it. "Here's your applesauce." Sherry stood her up from her chair and led her, shuffling, into the bathroom and then back to her bed.

"You're ready for the marathon, Mom," I said.

"She's a little better, Mr. Rosenfeld," declared Alma, as she invariably did, ladling up dinner.

Chick Budnitz came in about eight, assured himself by a glance that my mother was beyond his ministration, and sat down with us for lemon pie. He looked crushed. I felt sorry for him. She was wasting, he said, "living off capital." A low cough came from her room. "She could last a week."

A *week*, I thought to myself, at once glowering at my focus on my own relief and convenience. I did not want to wait.

The heavy flow of unscheduled visitors that began the next morning indicated that her Berkshire friends were aware of her decline. Sherry put on her lipstick and red robe and sat her in the lounge chair, and she received people with a faint smile as though she had a deeper problem on her mind.

Pat Hart, a retired social worker who'd taken pains to develop individual friendships with different Rosenfelds, bubbled for a while about her own doings in a monologue thoughtfully designed to spare my mother the need to respond.

Lee Cooperman, who had arrived in the Berkshires "only" in 1968, said to my mother, "I love you, Beth," and shortly left the room. Downstairs, she told me she and her husband Martin, a Stockbridge psychiatrist, had visited my father the night before he died and had seen in him the symptoms now visible in my mother. She recalled that my father had summoned the Coopermans on an earlier Sunday afternoon to announce that he had cancer.

Nat Horwitt, New York adman turned Stockbridge farmer, sat uneasily at bedside for a while. I went out with him. He observed that the Rosenfeld family was a close one and scooted out to his car to bring back a flat briefcase suitable for protecting a fragile eighty-year-old family scrapbook I'd been scanning.

Pat Hart was still there. I said to her that the period of dying had probably been easier for us than for most, because we were a close family and because my father had had enough money to ease what strains money can ease in such a situation.

She replied, "Others know tenderness, too."

At nine that night, when I'd already turned off the outside lights, a knock sounded. It was Court McDermott, head of the ski school at Bousquet's and the person who'd taught my mother (at age fifty) to enjoy skiing. He was coming not as a close friend but simply as someone in the community who'd liked her a lot.

I said I thought my mother's will had begun to fade when her husband died.

He replied that his father, an alcoholic, had willed his own death by a three-week binge. "Beth is a brave lady," he said.

Syd Pincu came the next day, gazing at my mother as

though to store up the sight against future time alone. Like my father, her husband had been a creative person (an architect) who, though long diverted into storekeeping, had kept his interest in his creative field. Syd had shared with my mother a lively interest in cultural exploration. She recalled how the two of them, preparing once to dabble in transcendental meditation, had been scolded out of it by my father. We laughed.

Bob Maislen, a pediatrician, dropped by, ever the sympathetic counselor. "It's hard to imagine how a sick person feels," he said to me. "She has no more energy to focus outside herself. What is she thinking? Perhaps anxiety. Perhaps there's metastasis (cancer spreading) in the brain."

Bea Mintz telephoned. Faulty brain surgery had left her mind sharp but her body dull twenty-five years ago. Had I told my mother of the death of Ruth Maeder, the friend who'd recently died? No. "That's good. Don't tell her, the poor thing."

Rex Fall, my father's *Eagle* crony, presented a single white chrysanthemum. "A lovely flower for a lovely lady," he said.

I could not pretend to be other than profoundly moved by these and other calls. They were heartcatching. Indeed, through the sentiment revealed in them I gained an extra respect for the quality of my parents' lives. The family had rejected the viewing of "remains" at a funeral home, but the paying of last respects to the living at the family home struck me as a practice far worthier of being enshrined as a universal custom. I recalled that I had sometimes stayed away from a friend's deathbed out of apprehension that a call might be regarded as an intrusion. But such calls—or letters written sooner to the dying rather than later to the survivors—are not intrusions but gifts. One does not necessarily have to choose in such situations between sharing while life remains and supporting after death has come, but if one does, my own choice is clear.

As I had rifled my mother's memory, I rifled my father's files for odd items not encountered before. It was a magpie's haul. A letter from his father, written in 1904 while he was "traveling" for a clothing house, reported a "peculiar dream" to be explained upon his arrival home from Little Falls, Minnesota. A second letter, written from St. Cloud, said about my father's fugitive brother Zeno, "He has got spirit enough, even if it's evil, to give each one of us a fling or a dig. I pocket mine gracefully. The Book is closed." There were World War I army papers and passes and an obituary of his father's spinster sister Kathinka, whose deathbed conversion had produced "the first instance on record in this city of the funeral of a Jewish person being held from a Catholic church."

In a tattered *Scribner's* of October 1927 my father was credited with coining "clairaudition," akin to clairvoyance, and in the January 1928 issue two previous users of that word were named. He had kept a clipping of an *Eagle* social note he'd planted which identified "Mr. and Mrs. Homer Pidgeon [*sic*] and daughter Cally (*callipygian*, according to Webster's, means having shapely buttocks) of Lower Montclair" as his overnight guests, and a letter quoting an *Eagle* editor as saying about his first music review, "The ending's pretty far from the beginning." There were copies of dozens of letters to editors, most of them dispatched either in defense of Israel or in criticism of the advertising and marketing practices of chain stores. He'd written to *Reader's Digest* that although Nestle's and Sara Lee had taken ads on consecutive pages, their merger "ain't Nestle Sara Lee so." I took an indulgent view of these suggestive bits and trivial pieces. They were of the man.

By Sunday my mother was untying moorings. To Becky, whom I put on the phone from Washington, she said, "Hello, darling" with startling clarity, then sank back exhausted.

"Mrs. Rosenfeld," said Sherry, asking in a way precluding a nod, "does your swimming pool open in May or June?"

A long pause, a knitting of brows. "June."

Alice McNiff, a Stockbridge friend who'd cut short her winter in Mexico, arrived, and my mother could only lift her hand, large-looking and loose on her swizzle-stick wrist.

I had caught the sniffles and asked myself briefly if I

should keep a distance. Then I realized the absurdity of the caution and said out loud, "Oh, what the hell." My mother did not stir. The sighs of breathing and occasional slow coughing replaced words.

Monday night I went into her room after dinner to say good night. I thought she was asleep but she murmured back the words. The picture was sharp of my hesitation in my last moment with my father. I took an instant vow not to let pass the opportunity to say, for the first time, perhaps for the last time, what I most wanted to say to her. "I love you," I said, bending close. She raised a hand.

She was choking on Tuesday and we summoned Budnitz to draw a sticky membrane from her mouth and throat. Her eyes took on a severe hurt look. I was feeling cooped up. Ron Goldfarb had offered to fly up from Washington to play tennis or otherwise assist in distraction. For a minute I wanted to call him.

Jayn and her family arrived. I drifted off. I'd found a photo of my father's old family house on Robbins Avenue and went out to see if the place was still there. It was gone but I could position myself across the street on the spot from which the photo had been taken and see that the old houses on either side were there.

Back at 173, someone who hadn't heard of my mother's condition called and asked to speak with her. I said she was sleeping.

About ten that night Jayn and I slipped in to say good night.

She raised her hand and said, "Hi."

Jayn's family and Alice filled the second-floor bed-rooms. I moved to the attic bedroom and awoke in the predawn darkness of Thursday, March 25. It was 4 A.M.

As I later learned, Sherry, from her bed a few feet from my mother's, had heard her shift restlessly and had turned on her flashlight just in time to see my mother raise both arms into the air. To stretch? To appeal? To surrender? It was 4 A.M.

I lay awake, straining for telltale sounds.

Dawn came: a soft day, some haze.

Shaving, over the sound of the running water, I heard footsteps on wooden stairs.

Jayn appeared at the door barefoot in her nightgown and said softly, "She's dead."

Both of us were caught in amusement at the spectacle of me receiving this news while standing in my underwear with lather still smeared on half my face. I touched her arm.

In a few minutes I was in my mother's room. The covers were drawn to her neck and her head was small on the pillow. "I love you," I said, kissing the cool cheek.

So, I said to myself, that's it. There was no sadness. The major purpose remaining to her life of seventy years had been taken away by the death of her husband five months earlier. She had made as much of an effort to find a new configuration for her life as her cancer had permitted. Her period of succumbing had brought back to her a fitting measure of the affection and attention she had conferred on others. This woman who did not know herself where she had been born, who had been uprooted and torn in her own beginnings, had put down roots and had spun her own ties and knew exactly where she was dying. She had died calmly. I met her death calmly. The transition from one generation to the next was done. I felt the world was in balance.

Jerry Seigel, my sister's husband, was quietly with us. Chick Budnitz was there. "That damn cancer kills a lot of people," he said. Alice McNiff came in and went out to keep Jayn's and Jerry's two daughters occupied in their room while the funeral home crew arrived and zipped the body in a purple bag and twisted and tilted the stretcher down the stairs. Jayn had already selected burial clothes, a wool dress my mother had bought on a European vacation and her favorite pearls. She and I started making calls. Others arrived to weave for us the now familiar pattern by which the community partici-pates in the ritual of loss.

After breakfast, I drove upstreet to see Jesse Spector, the cancer specialist. Young, self-confident, and mod—qualities my mother had liked in him—he had me tail him to the barbershop where he'd scheduled a haircut appointment, and we talked through her illness there. After my week's immersion, he was refreshingly profes-sional and sharp. He regretted, he said, having moved to Pittsfield so recently (the previous year) that he did not have occasion to know my mother except as a patient. I studied his hair on the floor.

Barbara and the children were there by the end of the afternoon. She fixed me with a direct gaze that mercifully shut everything else out, just for a moment. The kids tendered brief hugs. We settled two of them into my mother's bedroom, which Jayn had dubbed the "new TV room." I could not have stayed there but the kids didn't blink. Jerry made drinks. Alma beamed at the prospect of feeding a dozen people.

I raised a toast: "Mommy would have liked to see this table full of children and grandchildren and friends."

The kids clinked milk glasses against our wine.

And later Barbara sat on my lap and, with Jayn and Jerry, we began sifting out the last days. I felt my mother had died long ago.

Rarely assembled in full strength, the four of us Rosenfeld children, with spouses, gravitated to the yard in the sun the next morning and stood around talking, catching up and moving on, generating a nice comradeship. My sister Jayn (with her husband Jerry), my brothers Peter (with Lucy) and Rick (with Gillian), I (with Barbara)—we had all made our professional ways, married fortunately, become parents of healthy children and, collectively as much as any family, I supposed, kept in reasonable touch with our parents and each other. I could not help reflecting that we were our parents' children, their reflection as well as their pride, indebted to them, stamped by them. We are all strong adults and we can all walk without our parents, I thought. If our family kinetics were more complex than many outsiders suspected, then on this day I was prepared to let the community view stand unchallenged as a mark of respect to them. Some of our total of eleven children—no less "grandchildren" for having lost their grandparents—rocketed around the yard.

Only the two oldest of the eleven, Dave and Becky, were going to the funeral. This time there was no music. The rabbi's eulogy centered on my mother's community service. It ended with a reading of one of the quotations, from Hudson Maxim, that my father had chosen for his own funeral:

> "And when—if ever—I awake
>   In a celestial sphere,
> I ask no greater happiness
>   Than that she gives me here."

Again the ungainly wheeling out of the casket, which was covered by a cascade of roses grown by the same friend who'd prepared a funeral display for my father. Again the procession to the Pittsfield Cemetery. My father's grave was hidden by a cloth on which had been piled the dirt, itself covered, dug out for my mother's grave. I warmed thinking that she would again be next to her husband. More than missing her, I thought of her fondly. I had received from them the means to build a life of my own. I had given them a life of my own which they had respected, and a flow of concern—of different qualities at different times—over the years. The bargain of the generations, I judged, had been fairly kept. They had cared for us, we for them, and now we were caring for children of our own. "Yisgadal . . ." The Kaddish, the prayer for the dead, began. I shredded the petals of a rose from the coffin onto the grave.

For the memorial service at home, a candle in a glass jar was lit under the mantel on which the empty jar of my father's candle sat.

I asked my mother's older sister Miriam to think back about her childhood. At age twelve and a half ("I looked sixteen"), Miriam had dropped out of the eighth grade to work as a stock clerk at Bonwit's, she told me. From her weekly pay of $3.50 she brought 25 cents each for candy, to my mother and her twin, in the orphanage they'd been placed in. They so hated the place they cried the nights through. Finally Miriam convinced a guardian uncle to move them to a foster home, though it cost more.

My mother's friend of fifty years' standing, Fannie Cohen, leaned into another reminiscence about her early Zionist leanings. She recalled that on a trip to Europe my mother had met a Palestine-bound engineer who had asked her to accompany him.

"As a secretary or as a pal?" I asked.

Fannie's eyes crinkled. "As a secretary! But Francie wouldn't let her go."

I grinned, finding it not in the slightest irreverent to imagine that a shrunken yellow-skinned woman not yet an hour in her grave could have had as a young woman a life of her own.

People drifted out into the pleasant early-spring afternoon, the kind of day on which my parents would have sallied forth on a four-mile walk.

Only Pat Hart, unaware that Jews don't mourn on the Sabbath, showed up that night (Friday). She regrouped easily and we gave her a drink and one of my mother's coats. The distribution of her personal things to her personal friends had already been cheerfully begun. In this sharing, as it happened, Barbara, who wears the same size that my mother wore, came out especially well. For months afterwards, it successively startled and delighted me to see the younger form in a sweater or dress in which my mind's eye perceived my mother first.

We had to decide what to do with the Pittsfield house. Everyone realized it was not so much a property question as a matter of the future shape of the family. For without my parents holding the center, none of us could be certain just what kind of a family we would continue to be. Could we somehow keep the house for weekends or vacations, or for the eventuality that someone might want to move to Pittsfield or retire there? Fleetingly, I hoped so. But the size, sort, location, and expense of the house had to be factored, plus the differing circumstances and interests of the four children.

The equation was abruptly done. The necessary large and equal commitment by each of the four of us simply was not forthcoming. It was sentimental, I conceded, to have expected otherwise. We would keep the house just until the following summer, when a concert in memory of our parents had already been scheduled in the chamber music hall on South Mountain, on the far side of the mountain. Feeling suddenly empty, I went straight to the phone and made reservations to fly back to Washington the next day.

I slept poorly and woke up blue. Two Jehovah's Witnesses came to the door. Full of my father's anger at their presumption of the superiority of their religion over mine, I snapped at them foully—to my dismay, upsetting my sister with my fury.

Alice McNiff drove us to the Hartford airport in her camper. I pleaded fatigue and shut my eyes, coming alert only when she related to us a fantastic story about a California family she had known.

The family had planned a camping trip deep into Mexico. Their aged and well-loved mother, knowing she was dying, chose to go with them. Far from home, in her sleep, content, the old woman died. The family thought of the logistic and police hurdles they would have to cross if they reported the death to Mexican authorities. They chose instead to roll up the body in a newly bought rug atop their camper to bring it home for burial. But waking up in a desolate place on the road—still in Mexico—they discovered that *the rug and its contents had been stolen* while they slept. Another family consultation was conducted. They thought of the thieves and the police, of their own need to return home on a certain schedule, and of the feelings their mother had had in insisting on accompanying them on the trip. And they continued along the road.

The children were transfixed by this tale. I broke into a broad smile. We flew home.

TWELVE

Lessons

So what had I taken from the experience of escorting my parents to their death, in one son's fashion? For a person whose life has gone well, as mine has, there are few sustained passages in which emotional and psychological demands are made that take one far outside one's normal self. This was such a passage. I found it difficult but absorbing, positive, liberating. It made me think about my parents and, beyond that, about the possibilities of human existence in categories that had previously been strange to me. This is what ultimately defined the time of their dying.

In their individual approaches to life they displayed a resolution that made them heroic, in cultural anthropologist Ernest Becker's sense of striving for a sense of self-worth, and in their approaches to death they displayed a vulnerability that made them human: first denying death, then accepting it. They went as far as they could on their own strengths and then retreated—perhaps I had better say, advanced—into resignation to their mortality and into dependence on others, without a quaver of doubt or shame.

Karl Lipsky, who packs a gorgeous picnic basket, once said to me that anyone could go out in the woods and chew roots and berries like an animal. Similarly, to be strong, while strength is on tap, is no great trick. The test is to accept weakness with grace. This my parents did, especially my mother, though I must observe, in some mitigation of the implied comment on my father, that she did not have to absorb the powerful distraction of pain.

Before they contracted what I sometimes wryly thought of as "his and hers" cancers, I had had with them as an adult a relationship good enough to sustain long conservations and long stays, regular phone calls and mail, pleasure in their presence, and an absence of the sort of tensions that, I know, separate many of my contemporaries from their parents in all but formal and ritualistic ways. I was perhaps closer to my mother, who did not convey the aloofness and sense of sitting in judgment that my father could show, and who did not make his spoken and unspoken demands for accommodation to an idiosyncratic style. Especially after I married, my parents and I got along heartily. They loved my wife, adored our kids.

Yet it was not a particularly profound relationship. I had not explored explicitly with them either my deeper feelings about personal things, or theirs. Traditional roles were played. The grandchildren were often the link, or the buffer, between us.

Fortunately, there was enough in place to build on when their ordeal began. I doubt that great innovations of personality or relationship are possible during such a time. Neither parent nor child can suddenly overcome a lifetime's habit or default or incapacity. But they can move on from where they have been, and this is what we did. A good relationship became a special one. Feelings and degrees of feelings new to the family were excavated and shared. I could not shed all my awkwardness in the presence of emotional intimacy with my parents but I could diminish it to a point which allowed exchanges that glow for me still and that underlie an abiding sense of having completed an important journey.

I am telling only of my own situation but I could guess that my brothers and sister were partaking of the experience, too.

As a journalist, I am in the quintessentially modern

business, one that arises from the spread of society's attentions beyond the reach of the immediate clan, of trying to tell people who weren't there what it was like. Yet what I would say most emphatically about the death of a parent is that one must be there. Time and again I realized how futile it was to extract information or convey emotion at a distance.

"What's up? How are you?" I would ask my father and mother in turn on the phone. Rarely did I ever get back anything but a neutral, noncommittal nod. One had to be on the scene to find out how things were, and to become a part of things. Becoming such a part was, of course, the point of being there.

I do not think I was merely a voyeur. I have not gotten much more interested than I previously was in medicine, or specifically in cancer. But I do have the strong sense that a personal investment, starting with an investment in time, is an awfully good way to perform one's duty to a dying parent and to move beyond duty into the mutual benefits of caring and love.

A grown son or daughter with a career and family and distant home may not always feel attracted to the discharge of more than perfunctory duty in the dying situation. Yet, I like to think, against a certain amount of evidence to the contrary, that a child with a full life and a bustling family may be just the one to go "home" for a parent's departing. Such a child may already have the logistical and emotional capacity to fit even more activity into his life.

And if the raw time is simply not available, as often it will not be, then the need grows to make what time is available fruitful and rich. This requires an effort and a candor too seldom drawn on in one's daily routine.

To be the mature child of a dying parent, however, is more than an exercise in individual stretching. It is a community activity involving, as it does, not only oneself and one's family but friends and associates, even if they are not always aware of it. The sensation of impending loss makes one eager to reach out to others, on one level to relieve distress and on a deeper level to drink of the wisdom already in the community reservoir.

I would not minimize the value of the sympathy I received directly from various people around me, ranging from close friends who always were there, to office acquaintances who, reading my father's obituary, said a kind word as we passed in the corridor. But I would draw particular attention to the certainty that one who is near a dying person will start learning a great deal about death from other people, close friends and casual acquaintances alike, who wish not just to lend an ear but to borrow one, to tell about how the death of their parents developed and what it meant to them.

I came to hear the silent click of the switch opening up the emotional currents of someone who had something to say about death. Such people, who are everyone, are everywhere. They are a fraternity. Sons or daughters just starting down death's road with their parents should know that they are there. They should be ready to exploit their lore, their prior knowledge of the terrain.

Waiting once at a neighborhood bus stop to go to the airport, I struck up a conversation with a black man, also waiting, who'd just finished up a yard job. Seeing my suitcase, he asked where I was headed. He said he had been sitting in a North Carolina jail on a trumped-up traffic charge when his mother had died, and had regretted to that day that he had not been permitted to attend her funeral. So it was.

But it is of course one's wife, or husband, and children on whom falls the principal burden of helping one find the new limits within which to make a family death an occasion for sharing rather than for self-contained anger or sorrow or, perhaps worse, for not much at all.

I have been speaking about experiencing a parent's death in one's middle years, when one will not only be comforted by wife and children but taught by them. What is taught is diverse. The process unlocks emotional combinations as thrilling as they are unexpected. They are there.

I would not claim that my family life was transformed. But I think it fair to say that my family, far from being cheated by my attention to the dying of my parents, gained by being drawn into a rich and complex generational process.

There was added to the mix in my mind, moreover, a

realization that the possibilities of relief or retreat in one direction had been cut off, and I had now to come to terms with the new fact that my own family offered the only subsequent possibility for rescue from straits of personal emergency. I think this adds a layer of emotional value even to family relationships that might have been thought to be more than acceptable before. And since the "lesson" of seeing one's parents die is to be open and to follow the heart, then it is only natural to explore whether that attitude cannot be further extended to spouse and children.

Certainly one is prepared to be more humble in the face of human dependency, other people's and one's own.

"Grow old along with me!," exulted Robert Browning, "The best is yet to be, / The last of life, for which the first was made" (*Rabbi Ben Ezra*). To which I would say, hmm. There is a sense in which for my parents the last of life was the best—the last years, minus one. But the very last—the final months, weeks, days—were not the best. They were difficult, painful, undignified, if by "dignity," a word flogged into near meaninglessness, is meant first of all a measure of seeming control over one's own destiny.

H. L. Mencken had it about right: "A man does not die quickly and brilliantly, like a lightning stroke; he passes out by inches, hesitantly and, one may almost add, gingerly." Not to say, cruelly.

In my parents' instance, this process went forth with a marked absence of accompanying doctrine, religious, psychic, or otherwise. Neither of them introduced any larger ideas about the meaning of death, or the lack of meaning. My father's allusion to a "celestial sphere," in which he might retrieve his wife's gift of happiness, was only a sentimental flourish. Considerations of a hereafter, and the agency by which that state is experienced, the soul, may sustain some dying people, or terrify them, but my parents approached death as though it were a blank.

They did so out of sturdy habit and love of life and out of Jewish doctrine, which posits, or so most Jews believe, not a hereafter but what one might call a here-now. I read three or four books on "the Jewish way of death." They did not address death as such. They discussed the customs and concepts by which bereaved people are comforted and their allegiance to faith and community secured. Typically, the Kaddish, the mourning prayer, does not mention death; it is a survivor's pledge of Jewish continuity.

In precisely that spirit of affirming life, Jewish impulses and values flooded my parents' years. It was these which led them to plan for death, by making sure they did what they wanted to do while they lived, and on a more procedural level, by preparing as best they could for old age and illness, for the disposition of their bodies and their assets, and so on.

Under the influence of their example, I am making similar plans. I feel more intensely about the need for self-expression—not self-indulgence, I trust, but enjoying family and friends, digging deeper into work and play, trying to master more of my own time and my own times. When I have a particularly nasty or unnecessary fight with one of my children, for instance, then I may register the depressing thought that it is the best part of my life that I am allowing to trickle out here. Within weeks of my father's death, after years of procrastination, I made a will. For the first time, I undertook to pay systematic attention to my health, especially my diet. I thought hard about tennis.

Perhaps because my parents lived long lives, I did not develop a particular passion about cancer research. I do support such research, which should focus more on the causes, especially the environmental causes, of the cancers that will cut down young and middle-aged people in our increasingly chemicalized society, and less on the "cure" of cancers that take old people—if there is a "cure." My parents' cancers did not so much interrupt or shorten as end their lives. Neither they nor I regarded the disease as unnatural or unfair in itself. Statistically, they were going to die at that age of *something*.

What did come to trouble me greatly, however, was the cost of dying. Various health plans picked up almost all of the thousands of dollars of my parents' expenses for hospitalization and medical care. Home care, and the providing of their own chosen home setting for dying, they covered themselves. I would not have wanted it any other way.

Yet the health plans, public and private, cannot conceivably cover the costs of the increasing number of people who are living a long time and then dying slow, expensive deaths. The personal circumstances of many or most of these people obviously do not put within their means the comfortable options available to my parents.

The changing age profile of the American population sounds its own warning. The number of people sixty-five and over was 3.1 million in 1900, 9 million in 1940, and 20.1 million in 1970, and is expected to reach 31 million in the year 2000. Every year an extra 300,000 to 400,000 Americans are being added to the total making a claim on the resources available to that part of the population closest to death.

In earlier times, there was neither the medical knowledge to sustain long lives nor the expectation that the economic costs of aging would somehow be manageable. But now the medical knowledge is there, and so is the expectation that someone, in the last resort the government, will pick up the tab. The advance of knowledge has created one set of dilemmas centering on the extent to which technology should be used to mediate biological processes. The rising expectations of governmental cost-sharing are creating another set of dilemmas centering on the question of whose illnesses or what ill-nesses should be cared for when resources are insuf-ficient to cover them all.

This is essentially a political question, involving deci-sions by the government on the funding of particular kinds of research and care. I fear it has the potential, if not carefully managed, to induce real bitterness and divisiveness into an activity—health services in general, services for the aging and dying in particular—where consensus ought to prevail. I am glad that the dying of my parents never strayed into this political thicket. But the rest of us cannot expect to be equally fortunate.

Yet another effect of such "politicization" of death will surely be, I believe, to put a premium on values which can only be nourished within the family circle. In a fashion, the elements that make life "modern"—technology, urbanization, crowding, change of different sorts—draw people away from a direct concern with each other. Death can still draw people back. As my parents died, for instance, I felt relieved that our chil-dren were learning that death is something other than the detached, meaningless act it so often is portrayed as being on the shows they watch on television.

The essential problem of modern life on the daily level, as I see it, is to set up an appropriate balance be-tween public or political or technological demands, and the imperatives of one's private life. The context of a parent's dying can help one to restore that critical balance. It can let a grown son or daughter make a fresh calibration of the things that are important personally. It can open emotional channels and give a larger notion of one's possibilities as a child, as a parent, as a partner in a marriage, as a friend, as a member of a community and a citizen of the society beyond.

The chances of setting and holding a new values "ratchet" are, I would argue, better at age forty-three than, say, at thirty-three or twenty-three. Of course there is a cost: the cost of distress and loss. Some people are neither energized by it nor able to recover from it. But, I think, I am not one of them.

A terror of death dominates the human personality and forces all of us into various flights or exertions or beliefs in order to avoid being paralyzed in life, psychoanalysts say. Yet people who are in fact dying have no place to go—that is, no new place to go, no place where they have not already gone. Either they have acquired the emotional maturity to cope with what Ernest Becker called man's "earthly condition," the realization that he is unique among creatures but doomed to die, or they have not.

My parents, I believe, coped with their earthly condition. They did this in their respective manners, partly mutually, through the span of their lives. That is not what was stated in their obituaries or in other tributes but it is to me their final measure.

Whether a son can so emulate his parents is more

than a matter of intent or desire. It is a matter of all one's capacities, which flow only in incomplete and uncertain part from one's inheritance and which are only partially at one's conscious beck and call. Yet I must hope that, in the face of a like terror of death, I can respond in my life with the fullness and dignity that were at their command. To aspire to less would be to pay them less than their due.